Advances in Understanding Advocacy and Improving Policy Practice Education

A perennial issue in social work is the lack of clear evidence showing how to be a successful advocate and how to create enthusiasm among students for policy practice. Researchers are now applying theory to understand better the topics of effective social work advocacy and policy practice. The results of testing conceptual models with carefully gathered evidence are beneficial, helping us to advance our knowledge more quickly than merely collecting descriptions of case studies that remain unintegrated into a larger context. Improvements in understanding how to conduct effective advocacy emerge, helping practitioners to be more successful in their advocacy efforts. Similarly, bringing evidence and data to teaching methods improves confidence in their applicability to more than one course or institution. Readers of this book will discover how to be more effective policy practitioners as well as more engaging instructors by focusing on theories and evidence which demonstrate successful advocacy and teaching.

This book was originally published as a special issue of the *Journal of Policy Practice*.

Richard Hoefer is Roy E. Dulak Professor for Community Practice Research at the School of Social Work, University of Texas at Arlington, TX, USA. He directs the Center for Advocacy, Nonprofit, and Donor Organizations (CAN-DO) and the School's Professional Development Program. He also edits the *Journal of Policy Practice*.

Advances in Understanding Advocacy and Improving Policy Practice Education

Recent applications of theory and evidence

Edited by
Richard Hoefer

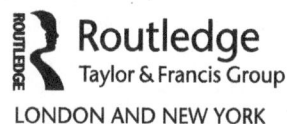

LONDON AND NEW YORK

First published 2016 by Routledge

2 Park Square, Milton Park, Abingdon, Oxfordshire OX14 4RN
711 Third Avenue, New York, NY 10017

Routledge is an imprint of the Taylor & Francis Group, an informa business

First issued in paperback 2018

Copyright © 2016 Taylor & Francis

All rights reserved. No part of this book may be reprinted or reproduced or utilised in any form or by any electronic, mechanical, or other means, now known or hereafter invented, including photocopying and recording, or in any information storage or retrieval system, without permission in writing from the publishers.

Notice:
Product or corporate names may be trademarks or
registered trademarks, and are used only for identification and explanation without intent to infringe.

British Library Cataloguing in Publication Data
A catalogue record for this book is available from the British Library

ISBN 13: 978-1-138-65125-8 (hbk)
ISBN 13: 978-0-367-02384-3 (pbk)

Typeset in Garamond
by RefineCatch Limited, Bungay, Suffolk

Publisher's Note
The publisher accepts responsibility for any inconsistencies that may have arisen during the conversion of this book from journal articles to book chapters, namely the possible inclusion of journal terminology.

Disclaimer
Every effort has been made to contact copyright holders for their permission to reprint material in this book. The publishers would be grateful to hear from any copyright holder who is not here acknowledged and will undertake to rectify any errors or omissions in future editions of this book.

Contents

Citation Information vii
Notes on Contributors ix

Introduction – Princess Wants a Dog Park: Using Theory and Evidence to Understand Advocacy and Improve Policy Practice Education 1
Richard Hoefer

1. Why Do Social Workers Become Policy Actors? 7
   Shiran Lustig-Gants and Idit Weiss-Gal

2. Leaning Out: Exploring Organizational Advocacy Activities From an Open Systems Perspective 27
   Lauri Goldkind

3. Identifying Attributes of Relationship Management in Nonprofit Policy Advocacy 48
   Nicole Ruggiano, Jocelyn Devance Taliaferro, Frank R. Dillon, Ted Granger, and Jessica Scher

4. Advocacy Tactics and Policy Outcomes of Sex Offender Rights Organizations 67
   Erin Comartin

5. NASW Involvement in Legislative Advocacy 92
   David Beimers

6. Human Rights and the Social Work Curriculum: Integrating Human Rights into Skill-Based Education Regarding Policy Practice Behaviors 111
   Julie A. Steen and Mary Mann

7. Civic Engagement and Civic Literacy Among Social Work Students: Where Do We Stand? 128
   Mary E. Hylton

8. Solving Current Social Challenges: Engaging Undergraduates in Policy Practice 144
   Margaret Sherraden, Baorong Guo, and Christine Umbertino

9. Embracing Applied Policy Practice: A Case Study From a Robust BSW Program 169
   Elizabeth Twining Blue and Lynn Amerman Goerdt

Index 183

Citation Information

The chapters in this book were originally published in the *Journal of Policy Practice*, volume 14, issue 3–4 (July–December 2015). When citing this material, please use the original page numbering for each article, as follows:

Introduction
Princess Wants a Dog Park: Using Theory and Evidence to Understand Advocacy and Improve Policy Practice Education
Richard Hoefer
Journal of Policy Practice, volume 14, issue 3–4 (July–December 2015), pp. 165–170

Chapter 1
Why Do Social Workers Become Policy Actors?
Shiran Lustig-Gants and Idit Weiss-Gal
Journal of Policy Practice, volume 14, issue 3–4 (July–December 2015), pp. 171–190

Chapter 2
Leaning Out: Exploring Organizational Advocacy Activities From an Open Systems Perspective
Lauri Goldkind
Journal of Policy Practice, volume 14, issue 3–4 (July–December 2015), pp. 191–211

Chapter 3
Identifying Attributes of Relationship Management in Nonprofit Policy Advocacy
Nicole Ruggiano, Jocelyn Devance Taliaferro, Frank R. Dillon, Ted Granger, and Jessica Scher
Journal of Policy Practice, volume 14, issue 3–4 (July–December 2015), pp. 212–230

Chapter 4
Advocacy Tactics and Policy Outcomes of Sex Offender Rights Organizations
Erin Comartin
Journal of Policy Practice, volume 14, issue 3–4 (July–December 2015), pp. 231–255

Chapter 5
NASW Involvement in Legislative Advocacy
David Beimers
Journal of Policy Practice, volume 14, issue 3–4 (July–December 2015), pp. 256–274

CITATION INFORMATION

Chapter 6
Human Rights and the Social Work Curriculum: Integrating Human Rights into Skill-Based Education Regarding Policy Practice Behaviors
Julie A. Steen and Mary Mann
Journal of Policy Practice, volume 14, issue 3–4 (July–December 2015), pp. 275–291

Chapter 7
Civic Engagement and Civic Literacy Among Social Work Students: Where Do We Stand?
Mary E. Hylton
Journal of Policy Practice, volume 14, issue 3–4 (July–December 2015), pp. 292–307

Chapter 8
Solving Current Social Challenges: Engaging Undergraduates in Policy Practice
Margaret Sherraden, Baorong Guo, and Christine Umbertino
Journal of Policy Practice, volume 14, issue 3–4 (July–December 2015), pp. 308–332

Chapter 9
Embracing Applied Policy Practice: A Case Study From a Robust BSW Program
Elizabeth Twining Blue and Lynn Amerman Goerdt
Journal of Policy Practice, volume 14, issue 3–4 (July–December 2015), pp. 333–346

For any permission-related enquiries please visit:
http://www.tandfonline.com/page/help/permissions

Notes on Contributors

Lynn Amerman Goerdt is Assistant Professor in Social Work at the University of Wisconsin–Superior, Superior, Wisconsin, USA.

David Beimers is Associate Professor in the Department of Social Sciences, Minnesota State University, Mankato, Minnesota, USA.

Erin Comartin is Assistant Professor in the Department of Sociology, Anthropology, Social Work & Criminal Justice, Oakland University, Rochester, Michigan, USA.

Jocelyn Devance Taliaferro is Associate Professor in the Department of Social Work, North Carolina State University, Raleigh, North Carolina, USA.

Frank R. Dillon is Associate Professor in the Division of Counseling and Psychology, School of Education, University at Albany – State University of New York, Albany, USA.

Idit Weiss-Gal is Associate Professor at the Bob Shapell School of Social Work, Tel Aviv University, Tel Aviv, Israel.

Shiran Lustig-Gants is a Researcher in the Welfare Department, Rishon LeZion, Israel.

Lauri Goldkind is Associate Professor at the Graduate School of Social Service, Fordham University, New York, USA.

Ted Granger is President of the United Way of Florida, Tallahassee, Florida, USA.

Baorong Guo is Associate Professor in the School of Social Work, University of Missouri–St. Louis, and Center for Social Development, Washington University, St. Louis, Missouri, USA.

Richard Hoefer is Roy E. Dulak Professor for Community Practice Research at the School of Social Work, University of Texas at Arlington, Texas, USA.

Mary E. Hylton is Associate Professor in the School of Social Work, University of Nevada, Reno, Nevada, USA.

Mary Mann is an Instructor at the School of Social Work, University of Central Florida, Orlando, Florida, USA.

Nicole Ruggiano is Associate Professor in the School of Social Work, Robert Stempel College of Public Health and Social Work, Florida International University, Miami, Florida, USA.

NOTES ON CONTRIBUTORS

Jessica Scher is Public Policy Director at the United Way of Miami-Dade, Miami, Florida, USA.

Margaret Sherraden is Professor at the School of Social Work, University of Missouri–St. Louis, and Center for Social Development, Washington University, St. Louis, Missouri, USA.

Julie A. Steen is Associate Professor in the School of Social Work, University of Central Florida, Orlando, Florida, USA.

Elizabeth Twining Blue is a PhD student in Social Work at the University of Wisconsin–Superior, Superior, Wisconsin, USA.

Christine Umbertino is a Researcher at the Brown School of Social Work, Washington University, St. Louis, Missouri, USA.

INTRODUCTION

Princess Wants a Dog Park: Using Theory and Evidence to Understand Advocacy and Improve Policy Practice Education

RICHARD HOEFER

School of Social Work, University of Texas at Arlington, Arlington, Texas, USA

Elizabeth Covington had an issue that she wanted the Town Council to address. Her dog, named Paddy, needed a leash-free dog park nearby and there was not one (Hundley, 2014; Roark, 2014). While it isn't clear all the initial steps Ms. Covington took to promote her idea, several steps can be found in the public record. It appears she worked with other citizens to create momentum for the idea and to help influence elected officials, including bringing a petition with at least 400 signatures to the town council (date unclear). As early as February 2010, someone created a Facebook page to promote the idea. The Facebook page is called "Princess Wants a Dog Park in Flower Mound" and a website called www.princesswantsadogpark.com.

On October 9, 2013, at 2:22 p.m., local news reported that the project was funded, a location was found and it would be completed by spring, 2014. The project would cost about $600,000, including amenities such as vinyl-covered chain link fencing with separate areas for large and small dogs, a restroom for people, dog waste containers, etc. A disc-golf park was also proposed as part of the project but this raised the cost to over $1,000,000. (NBC DFW News, 2013, Oct. 9).

Five months later, on March 19, 2014, Town Council voted to look at a different location for the project. The price was now expected to cost between $700,000 and $800,000. The planned location had to be changed at least twice because of complaints by people who lived near proposed locations, working through their homeowners' associations and on their own. Eleven locations were considered before one was found that was not nixed by costs or residential opposition to increased traffic and congestion in residential areas (Hundley, 2014; Roark, 2014).

In September 2014, another meeting was held by the Town Council. At that time, the originator of the idea, Elizabeth Covington, stated: "I've been patient, worked with the system and I've been nice. It's time to pick up a shovel, dig some dirt, and get moving" (Cobb, 2015).

Three months later, in December 2014, Town Council decided on a location and, combining at least two planned improvement projects, renamed the project from "the Dog Park" to Heritage Park Phase II. It now includes full parking, installation of a pond, black vinyl chain link fence with concrete mow strips, hybrid Bermuda grass, irrigation, standard information signage, minimal landscaping, conduit for future lighting in the parking lot in the dog park. The project was to be put out to bid on April 7, 2015, to have a start construction date in May 2015, and an estimated completion date of June 2016 (Town of Flower Mound, 2015).

At its April 20, 2015, meeting, Town Council approved a bid for the dog park. On May 2, 2015, the Cross Timbers Gazette, covering Flower Mound and nearby towns, reported the project was about to start (Cobb, 2015).

This is a homely story, one that might not be considered at all important. At first glance, it is not at all relevant to the topic of policy practice for social workers. But I think it has the potential to be a teaching tool of the most important kind as well as something that will help all of us write better, more vital, more interesting, and ultimately, more impactful journal articles.

Let's review: What happened during this five-years plus period?

A town council decided, at the urging of a number of its residents, to build a dog park costing close to $800,000. Certain aspects of the plan (such as a kiosk building, shade areas, and lighting) were not approved at the current time, although infrastructure to make them possible in the future was included in the project.

Two other things happened. The website www.princesswantsadogpark.com became inactive, as did the Facebook page with the same name. More unfortunately, sometime in September 2014, the dog who wanted a dog park in Flower Mound, Princess, crossed the rainbow bridge to be in an eternal no-leash dog park. I find this entire saga fascinating because I want to be able to answer a question:

How did this dog park "happen"?

A basic answer is something like this: Citizen input and advocacy for the dog park started the process; citizen action to put the dog park in someone else's neighborhood delayed the project. No one objected to the park itself, just its location. In the end, despite initial misgivings about the cost, the plan as presented was approved, with delays in spending for certain amenities.

This basic answer is actually somewhat boring. It is really just a restatement of the earlier description that at least had some twists and turns to it. Instead, what I want to do is compare this story in a meaningful way to stories about dog parks being established across the country. More than that, I want to be able to compare this story to stories about municipal expenditures in Flower Mound and other towns. And, even more than that, I want to understand how policies get made—who is involved, how they are involved, when their involvement begins, what keeps them at it, how they react to defeats and setbacks.

I want to know who the people are who become advocates for dog parks, parks for people, social services for humans, tax breaks for billionaires, and every other type of policy.

There's so much more I want to understand, as well. How do people persuade other people—the people with the power to decide policy and money matters? What do decision makers look for when they are making a decision on policy? When is the system open to people of all types and with all levels of resources? When is it useful to work "inside the system" and when is it a waste of breath? When must we "take it to the streets"? How do policy areas differ from one another? How do different locations function similarly and what patterns hold true? When do advocates link up and when do they stay separate?

My goodness, I'm curious about this stuff—and it can all start with a story about a dog park in a community of fewer than 70,000 residents.

But—and this is important, so if you only remember one thing about this introduction (other than that Princess died before getting her dog park), remember this—the best way to really satisfy curiosity that extends beyond the bare facts is to employ a theory.

The Role of Theory in Advocacy Research

Kurt Lewin, father of social psychology, wrote in 1935 in the magnificent book, *A Dynamic Theory of Personality*, "There is nothing so practical as a good theory." (http://psychology.about.com/od/psychologyquotes/a/lewinquotes.htm).

First, let's review what a theory is. According to one definition: A theory presents a concept or idea that is testable. A theory is a fact-based framework for describing a phenomenon. Theories can be used to provide a model for understanding human thoughts, emotions, and behaviors (http://psychology.about.com/od/tindex/f/theory.htm).

For social policy, and advocacy, a theory should both describe behavior and predict it. A theory should allow us to focus on what to look at as well as to tell us under what conditions certain behaviors will occur. These predictions should be able to be made BEFORE you start looking. As an academic, a writer, and a journal editor, I want to see more use of theories from psychology, sociology, political science, policy studies, and more. This is important in the field of advocacy. If we are to become evidence-based in our advocacy practice, we need go beyond description of advocacy efforts to understanding the efforts and the outcomes and creating hypotheses about what works, with whom, and when.

We need to test hypotheses so that we are more capable and effective advocates ourselves. Even more important, we need to know what makes some advocacy successful and other advocacy unsuccessful so that we can teach and model what works to our students and the community at large. Social work, as a profession dedicated to advocacy for social justice, has to go beyond story telling to using stories to teach what works. What should our graduates do when, heartbreakingly, their clients need resources that are slated to be slashed?

What's Ahead?

The articles in this issue will help you as a scholar, educator, and/or practitioner to handle questions regarding how practitioners and educators can become better advocates and how to help students become skilled advocates as well. Some authors use theories explicitly, while others have less obviously used a framework or set of ideas to structure their work. Yet each of these contributions adds something of value to our understanding of advocacy, advocates, and the teaching of advocacy in social work. Many of these papers were first presented at the Social Policy Conference held in San Antonio in May 2014. All of them are worthy of your time to digest thoroughly.

The first five articles focus on advocates and advocacy. "Why Do Social Workers Become Policy Actors?" by Shiran Lustig-Gants and Idit Weiss-Gal focuses on one of the key questions for the profession. The Policy Practice Engagement Framework, and its key components (Opportunity, Facilitation, and Motivation) provide a fertile approach to understanding the topic. Using this theory-based model, the authors are able to provide not only the answer to the title's question, but also can give some clear answers to the question of how we can promote more social workers to become policy actors. In this case, the theory is very practical!

Lauri Goldkind gives us a treat by using an open systems perspective to help us understand organizational advocacy activities. The particular strength of "Leaning Out: Exploring Organizational Activities From an Open Systems Perspective" is the use of the Competing Values Framework, a way to assess the impact of organizational culture on advocacy efforts. As with any framework, one manuscript doesn't cover all the elements, so there is room for others to continue using the same framework.

Nicole Ruggiano, Jocelyn Devance Taliaferro, Frank R. Dillon, Ted Granger, and Jessica Scher use an approach predicated on managing relationships between the advocate and the advocate's target. Based on previous knowledge that relationships are key to successful advocacy, the authors detail how this process works for human services administrators, using strategies centered on access, positivity, openness, sharing of tasks, networking, and assurances. Knowing which of these factors have an impact, and why, provides social work administrators a leap forward in their efforts to be successful advocates.

Erin Comartin, using interviews with leaders of organizations working with stigmatized groups, details effective and ineffective tactics used by these organizations. Dividing the organizations into those that are proactive and those that are reactive, Comartin gives us deep insights into which tactics result in more influence with policymakers. Providing this information on organizations working with clients who are looked down upon gives practitioners hope that positive change can be made for clients that many decision makers look down on.

David Beimers moves us from the individual social worker or administrator to the social worker's largest professional organization—the National Association of Social Workers. In what ways and to what extent does this institution involve itself in legislative advocacy? Is it possible to move it more in that direction? What theories might help us better understand the situation? The field of political science has many insights into organizational advocacy practices and the reasons for them. This piece has some interesting empirical elements that can add to our understanding, particularly if the reader supplies a strong theoretical understanding to them.

We next move to four articles focusing on advocacy and social work education. Julie A. Steen and Mary Mann show how the integration of human rights into the social work curriculum can be accomplished and discuss the benefits of doing so. Having this as a curriculum resource will be helpful to social work education programs across the United States and even beyond. Mary E. Hylton asks social work students basic questions regarding their levels of civic engagement and civic literacy. If, as many fear, social work students do not know about basic concepts of government policymaking, it is difficult to think that they will be active. This sample of students reported more volunteering in the arena of human services than being politically active. Hylton finds a connection between understanding the political system and being active in it. This may provide additional impetus for ensuring that social work students acquire basic civics knowledge before leaving higher education.

The final two articles approach strengthening policy practice within undergraduate social work education. Margaret Sherraden, Baorong Guo, and Christine Umbertino provide clear examples of ways to promote policy practice in this level of professional education. Elizabeth Twining Blue and Lynn Amerman Goerdt provide a case study of how one BSW program was able to embrace policy practice fully. These authors provide special insight into how the topics of policy practice and advocacy can be put into place early in a professional's educational journey. The benefits to the student, the profession, and our society are considerable.

Conclusion

It's my firm belief, backed by countless examples, that ordinary citizens, with no professional training or background in advocacy skills, can conduct multi-year campaigns to create change on the local level. I also believe that that social work students and professionals can overcome great barriers to achieving social justice. As educators, we in CSWE-accredited institutions must ensure our students are competent in advocacy. These articles help us in our work and assist us in standing strong for social justice causes.

REFERENCES

Cobb, D. (2015, May). Dog park coming to area. *The Cross Timbers Gazette*, p. A3.

Hundley, W. (2014, Mar. 19). Flower Mound council oks site for town's first dog park. Retrieved from http://www.dallasnews.com/news/community-news/lewisville-flower-mound/headlines/20140318-flower-mound-council-oks-site-for-town-s-first-dog-park.ece

NBC DFW News (2013, Oct. 9). Flower Mound to build off-leash dog park. Retrieved from http://www.nbcdfw.com/news/local/Flower-Mound-to-Build-Off-Leash-Dog-Park-227109151.html

Roark, C. (2014, Mar. 19). Flower Mound council approves location for dog park. Retrieved from http://starlocalmedia.com/theleader/flower-mound-council-approves-location-for-dog-park/article_f1ffe33c-ae28-11e3-819c-0019bb2963f4.html

Town of Flower Mound (2015, Mar. 31). Heritage Park Phase II dog park. Retrieved from http://www.flower-mound.com/index.aspx?NID=686

Why Do Social Workers Become Policy Actors?

SHIRAN LUSTIG-GANTS
Welfare Department, Rishon LeZion, Israel

IDIT WEISS-GAL
Bob Shapell School of Social Work, Tel Aviv University, Tel Aviv, Israel

The study examines factors related to social workers' involvement in policy practice by examining their engagement in legislative advocacy in Israel. Based on the three components of the Policy Practice Engagement Framework—opportunity, facilitation and motivation—the study focused upon a group of social workers who were actively involved in legislative advocacy as part of their professional job. In order to learn more about their features and the circumstances of their legislative advocacy, they were asked about their testimonies and were then compared to a group of social workers who have never participated in the deliberations of legislative committees. The sample consisted of 190 social workers evenly divided between the two groups. The findings underscore that the intersect of opportunity, facilitation, and motivation created a context that encouraged the involvement of social workers in a specific form of policy practice. The study findings emphasize the opportunity and facilitation components of the framework over the motivational.

The social work discourse in different countries regards policy-focused activities as a key component and critical dimension of social work practice (Cochran & Davis, 2012; CSWE, 2010, Greene & Knee, 1996; Jansson, 2014; NASW, 2010; Mendes, 2013). These activities, identified by a variety of terms, among them, "policy practice" (Cummins, Byers, & Pedrick, 2011; Ritter, 2013), "policy advocacy" (Mosley, 2013; Pierce, 2000), "cause advocacy"

(Hoefer, 2012) or "class advocacy" (Ezell, 1994; Pierce, 1984), are viewed as important professional endeavors aimed at furthering social justice, human rights, and social inclusion, and better addressing service users' difficulties and needs (Colby, 2008; Ellis, 2008; Hoefer, 2013).

Over the past three decades, a growing discussion on factors that either impede or promote social workers' involvement in policy-focused activities has emerged (Abramovitz, 1998; Ezell, 1991, 1993; Hoefer, 2013; Jacobson, 2001; Rocha, Poe, & Thomas, 2010). However, only a small number of studies sought to empirically examine those factors. Moreover, most of these focused on factors associated with social workers' political participation, which include partisan political activities, voting in elections, or volunteer work for a political party or a candidate for political office, all of which take place outside the social workers' work settings (Ezell, 1993; Hamilton & Fauri, 2001; Hartnett, Harding, & Scanlon, 2005; Ritter, 2007, 2008). These activities are clearly substantial and are potentially indicative of social workers' commitment to policy involvement. However, they can be best construed as facets of civic involvement and do not necessarily relate directly to social workers' professional activities. Indeed a very limited number of studies have attempted to better understand the engagement of social workers in, what Ezell (1994) termed, job-related advocacy. These policy-focused activities are an integral part of social workers' professional endeavors (i.e., they are undertaken in the context of the social worker's workplace). Activities include advising or lobbying policymakers with regard to policy issues related to the agency domain or to client groups, teaching clients advocacy skills, analyzing a policy or social problem on the organizational, local, or government levels, or giving testimony in legislative committees.

The aim of the study presented in this article was to enrich knowledge on factors related to social workers' involvement in policy-focused activities as an integral component of their professional role (termed here "policy practice") by examining their engagement in legislative advocacy. Distinctive from previous empirical work on policy practice, which has typically drawn upon case studies or self-reported engagement in policy practice, this study focused upon a group of social workers identified in a previous study as having been actively involved in legislative advocacy as part of their professional job as social workers (Gal & Weiss-Gal, 2011). More concretely, it concentrated upon those social workers who participated in at least three legislative committee meetings in the *Knesset* (Israel's parliament). In order to learn more about their features and the circumstances in which their engagement in legislative advocacy occurred, they were asked about their testimonies and were then compared to a group of social workers who have never participated in the deliberations of legislative committees.

CONCEPTUAL BASIS

The conceptual basis of the study is the Policy Practice Engagement (PPE) framework (Gal & Weiss-Gal, 2015). This framework draws upon diverse theoretical sources in order to shed light on the factors that influence social workers' involvement in policy practice in different policy arenas and national settings. More specifically, it seeks to explain *why* social workers engage in policy practice and *how* they tend to intervene in the policy process. The framework encompasses three interrelated but distinct components: Opportunity, Facilitation, and Motivation.

Opportunity refers to the degree to which policy formulation institutions are accessible to social workers seeking to influence the policy process. The framework underscores that social workers' policy practice is contingent upon institutional arrangements that exist in various phases of the policy formulation process and which determine formal and informal norms and rules. These norms and rules are crucial in that they influence the accessibility of this process to members of the social work profession (Mosley, 2013; Schneider & Netting, 1999). As it is contingent on context-specific norms and rules, *opportunity* varies between nations and between different policy formulation arenas and it can obviously change over time. In Israel, *Knesset* legislative committee sessions are relatively accessible to members of the public and, in particular, to stakeholders and to professionals with relevant knowledge (Rubinstein & Medina, 2005). In addition, civil servants are routinely invited to participate in meetings pertaining to their field of responsibility. As, by law, all senior officials dealing with social welfare are required to be qualified social workers, social workers enjoy comparatively high levels of opportunity to testify before legislative committees (Gal & Weiss-Gal, 2011; Weiss-Gal & Gal, 2014). A full examination of the degree to which social workers have an opportunity to engage in policy practice obviously requires a comparison of different policy arenas in a single national context or across countries. As this study focused upon a single policy arena in one country, it does not lend itself to a full-fledged exploration of the degree to which *opportunity* affected the engagement of social workers in policy practice. However, it was assumed that it would be possible to shed some light on the *opportunity* component by exploring the dynamics through which social workers accessed the legislative committees. In other words, the study sought to understand who initiated the social worker's appearance in the committees assuming that, if this was at the committee's behest (rather than that of the social worker), this would be indicative of the more active form that *opportunity* took in this case. *Opportunity* then was examined by determining the route by which the social workers were invited to the legislative committee deliberations—if it was at the initiative of the committee administration, the individual social worker, or the agency in which she or he was employed.

The *facilitation* component refers to the degree to which a social worker's workplace enables, and indeed encourages, policy practice. The assumption here is that organizational characteristics and culture will affect social workers' involvement in policy practice in that they will reflect the degree to which policy engagement is an acceptable form of social work practice and, if so, the form that this will take and who will engage in it. The fact that social workers tend to work in diverse welfare sectors will have a major impact in determining the degree to which they engage in policy practice (Ezell, 1994). On an aggregative level, the norms that determine acceptable professional behavior within each sector and the perceived legitimacy of interventions in the policy field are critical in this context and will influence the boundaries of permissible engagement in the policy arena. The public service ethos in a specific national setting will set the boundaries of policy practice for social workers who are government employees while arguably local government social workers will be influenced by place-specific guidelines (in addition to more universal directives and rules). Alternately, social workers employed by a range of nonprofits will operate under a different and presumably more diversified set of rules and norms.

It can also be assumed that social workers' specific role in an organizational hierarchy will have a facilitating impact upon their engagement in the policy arena. Often higher-ranking administrative roles will entail a greater role in policy formulation. Indeed, more advanced positions in this hierarchy will lead to greater exposure on the part of social workers in administrator roles to the policy process, to a greater willingness to devote time and effort to policy activities (Ezell, 1991), and to more demands by their employees to intervene in this arena (Weiss-Gal & Levin, 2010).

The current study thus examined two organizational features in facilitating social workers' engagement in legislative advocacy: sectoral affiliation (national government, local government, the nonprofit sector) and the social worker's role (administrative or not) within the organization.

The *motivation* component focuses on the motivation of individual social workers to engage in policy practice and includes both internal and external factors. Internal factors pertain to the values, capabilities, perceptions, and traits of the individual social worker (Ezell, 1994). Drawing on the Civic Voluntarism Theory (Verba, Schlozman, & Brady, 1995) which has been shown to be useful in studying social workers' political participation, the PPE framework identifies internal factors that help explain social workers' policy practice participation. These include personal resources, psychological engagement in politics, and recruitment networks that will induce individuals to participate in policy processes. External factors relate to elements in the social worker's professional environment that can encourage (or discourage) engagement in policy practice. These will typically include the professional discourse, activities of professional organizations and, in particular, social work education (Anderson & Harris, 2005; Tower & Hartnett, 2011; Zubrzycki & McArthur, 2004).

As such, *Motivation* was assessed by studying seniority, psychological engagement in politics, and policy practice training. The study focused on seniority as a proxy for the place of social workers' personal resources as a motivation source for engagement in policy practice. This was based on the assumption that seniority offers social workers a greater sense of job security and expertise in their field and thus those with more seniority will be more motivated to intervene in the policy process. They will also be more able to identify lacunae in their field and less hesitant to express their views regarding policies. Likewise, it was assumed that social workers with a higher level of psychological engagement in politics (political interest, political efficacy, and partisanship) will be more motivated to engage in policy practice. In addition, the study tested the assumption that policy practice training can play an important role in increasing social workers' engagement in policy practice. Finally, in cases in which social workers in the study group (as opposed to the committee administration or the agency) initiated their participation in the committee meetings, their justification for this was sought.

In sum, this study sought to enhance knowledge of the factors linked to social workers' involvement in policy practice by focusing upon a group of social workers who participated in three or more legislative committee meetings ("the study group"). After identifying a number of features of the circumstances in which the participation of the social workers in the legislative committee meetings took place, the study group was then compared to a group of social workers who did not participate in these meetings ("the comparison group").

More specifically the study addressed five questions:

1. What were the study group members' socio-demographic (age), professional and organizational features (seniority and role), and organizational affiliation (government, local, nonprofit) when they first participated in a legislative committee?
2. Did the study group members have a higher level of psychological engagement in politics than those in the comparison group?
3. Did the study group members have more policy practice training than those in the comparison group?
4. Are there differences in the general levels of policy practice engagement between social workers in the study group and those in the comparison group?
5. Who initiated the social workers' first committee appearance and their subsequent appearances, and did this vary with the social workers' organizational affiliation? In instances in which the social workers initiated their participation in the committee meeting, what motivated this?

METHOD

Sample

The sample consisted of 190 social workers evenly divided between the study and comparison groups. The study group consisted of social workers who participated in three or more legislative committee meetings during the 15th and 16th *Knesset* sessions (1999–2006). The comparison group consisted of social workers who had never participated in any legislative committee meeting.

The study group was constructed in three stages. First we obtained the names and organizational affiliation of 667 social workers identified in a previous study as participants in legislative committee deliberations (Gal & Weiss-Gal, 2011) and selected those 187 social workers who had attended at least three legislative committee meetings. Attending three or more meetings was assumed to be indicative of engagement in policy practice in this arena that was more than one-off. In the second stage, we sought contact information for 174 of the selected social workers. Their phone numbers and/or e-mail addresses were obtained from their workplaces, by Google searches and through the databases of the Ministry of Welfare and Social Services and various municipalities. In the third stage, we contacted the workers, explained the study, and asked them to participate in it. Ninety five agreed, a response rate of 54.5%.

The comparison group was drawn from a convenience sample of 178 social workers in a range of local, national, and nonprofit social welfare agencies throughout Israel. In each agency, we distributed the study questionnaire, which included a question asking if the respondent had ever participated in a legislative committee meeting. To create the comparison group we removed the 12 workers who answered this question positively. We also removed those social workers who had particularly limited working experience in order to reduce the gap between the seniority of the study group and the comparison group.

The demographic and professional features of the two groups, Chi square comparison and *t*-tests are presented in Table 1 (nominal variables) and Table 2 (interval variables).

As can be seen, no significant differences were found in gender, nationality, or specialization in BSW or MSW studies. About three quarters of the study participants were women and almost all were Jewish. With respect to specialization, at the BSW[1] level, somewhat over half did not have any specific specialization; about a third specialized in direct work with individuals and families; and about 10% specialized in community work. At the MSW

---

[1] A BSW is the degree required to receive a social work license in Israel. An MSW degree is an advanced practice or research degree.

TABLE 1 The Demographic and Professional Features of the Study and Comparison Groups (n,%) (N = 190)

Characteristic	Value	The study group (n = 95)		The comparison group (n = 95)		Total (n = 190)		χ^2
		N	%	N	%	N	%	
Gender	Female	74	77.9	67	70.5	141	74.2	1.34
	Male	21	22.1	28	25.8	49	25.8	
Nationality	Jewish	90	94.7	93	97.9	183	96.3	1.32
	Arabs	5	5.3	2	2.1	7	3.7	
Education	BSW only	6	6.3	26	27.4	32	16.8	15.03***
	MSW	89	93.7	69	72.6	158	83.2	
Specialization (BSW)	None	50	52.6	53	55.8	103	54.2	
	Direct work	30	31.6	36	37.9	66	34.7	4.49
	Macro practice	15	15.8	6	6.3	21	11.1	
Specialization (MSW)	Direct work	37	38.9	35	36.8	72	37.9	1.28
	None	32	33.7	39	41.1	71	37.4	
	Macro practice	26	27.4	21	22.1	47	24.7	
Organizational affiliation	Governmental	44	46.3	21	21.9	65	34	28.96***
	Nonprofit	36	37.9	25	26	61	31.9	
	Local	15	15.8	50	52.1	65	34	

***$p < .001$.

TABLE 2 Age and Seniority: Means, Standard Deviations, and t-Values

Characteristic	The study group (n = 95)		The comparison group (n = 95)		T
	M	SD	M	SD	
Age	56.62	8.98	44.75	9.15	8.04***
Seniority	28.2	9.12	16.98	10.09	9.02***

***$p < .001$.

level, some 40% specialized in direct practice and about a quarter specialized in community work.

Significant differences were found in age, social work degree, organizational affiliation, and seniority. The workers in the study group were about 10 years older than those in the comparison group. They were better educated, with more than 90% percent having an MSW degree, as opposed to somewhat over 70% of the comparison group. In organizational affiliation, the two groups were practically mirror images of one another. In the study group, around half were employed in a national government ministry, over a third in nonprofit (mostly advocacy) organizations, and about a fifth in local government. In the comparison group, over half worked in local government, about a fifth in a national government ministry, and about a quarter in nonprofits. Finally, the social workers in the study group had approximately 11 years more seniority than those in the comparison group.

ANCOVAs were performed to control for the significant differences in seniority, education, and age. Two-way MANOVAs were carried out to control for differences in organizational affiliation.

Instruments

The participants filled out a series of self-report questionnaires, most of which were filled out by both groups, though some were only relevant to the study group.

Questionnaires filled out by both groups. Demographic characteristics were ascertained by questions on gender and age.

Professional characteristics were ascertained by three questions asking 1. Social work degree (BSW/MSW); 2. Specialization during BSW and MSW studies; and BSW and MSW studies; 3. Years of social work experience (seniority).

Organizational features were queried by open questions with respect to the current time and (for the study group) the date of their first legislative committee meeting. For each point in time, respondents were asked to indicate their organizational affiliation and role. We then categorized their answers into three types of organizations (national government, local government, and nonprofits) and four roles: front line, team head, supervisor, and administrator.

Policy practice training was ascertained by one question: "To what extent did you learn how to influence policy during your social work studies (whether BSW, MSW, or continuing studies)?" Responses were made on a 5-point Likert scale ranging from 1 = not at all to 5 = to a large extent. The higher the score, the greater the exposure to ways of influencing policy during social work education.

Psychological engagement in politics was assessed by three variables: political interest and discussion, political efficacy, and partisanship. The scales were developed by Verba et al. (1995) and translated and modified to the Israeli context in a previous study (Teush, 2012).

Political interest and discussion was measured by two questions, each asked twice, once with respect to local politics, once with respect to national politics. The questions were: "How often do you discuss politics with friends, neighbors or relatives?" and "How interested are you in politics?" Answers were made on a 5-point Likert scale ranging from 1 (not at all) to 5 (to a large extent). Cronbach's alphas were acceptable: $\alpha = .82$ for local politics and $\alpha = .83$ for national politics. Two scores, the means of the two items, were calculated for each participant. The higher the score, the greater the social worker's interest in local/national politics.

Political efficacy was also measured by two questions, each asked twice, once with respect to local politics, once with respect to national politics. The questions were "How much attention do you think that a policy-maker(government minister, parliament member, senior official) would pay to a complaint regarding a government activity or policy that you brought to him or her?" and "How much influence do you think someone like you can have on government decisions?" The questions were answered on a 5-point Likert scale ranging from 1 (not at all) to 5 (to a large extent). Cronbach's alphas were acceptable: $\alpha = .65$ for the local level, $\alpha = .67$ for the national level. Two scores, the means on each factor, were calculated for each participant. The higher the scores, the greater the social worker's sense of political efficacy.

Partisanship was ascertained by one question: "To what extent do you feel a strong identification with a particular political ideology or political party?" Answers were made on a 5-point Likert scale ranging from 1 (not at all) to 5 (to a large extent). The higher the score, the greater the partisanship.

Engagement in policy practice was ascertained by one question asked twice, once with respect to the organization where the social worker was employed and again with respect to the national level. The question was "During your career as a social worker, to what extent have you engaged in activities aimed at changing a policy?" Answers were made on a 5-point Likert scale ranging from 1 (not at all) to 5 (to a large extent). Two scores were calculated for each respondent, one for engagement in organizational policy, the other for engagement in national policy. The higher the score, the greater the social worker's engagement in policy practice.

Questionnaires filled out only by the study group. We ascertained who initiated the social worker's participation in the committee meetings by way of two questions: "Who initiated your first committee testimony?" and "Who initiated most of your subsequent testimonies?" For each, the respondents were asked to choose the most accurate option: (a) The committee administrator asked me to participate; (b) The committee administrator asked my workplace for someone to participate; (c) My supervisor asked me to participate on his/her own initiative; and (d) My own initiative.

Reasons for initiating the participation were queried in an open question, "What were your reasons for initiating the testimony?" addressed to the respondents who had initiated their participation themselves. Content analysis was performed on the responses.

Procedure

Approval for the study was received from the Ethics Committee of the Hebrew University of Jerusalem. The data were collected between September 2012 and March 2013. All the study participants were informed that participation was voluntary and anonymous and gave their agreement to participate, either by phone or e-mail.

In the initial telephone calls to gather the study sample, the social workers who agreed to participate were asked whether they preferred to answer the questions by e-mail or telephone. Fifty-eight percent chose e-mail; 42% chose telephone. No significant differences were found in the responses to the study questions of those who answered by phone and those who answered via e-mail. The members of the comparison group were sent the study questionnaires by e-mail.

FINDINGS

In order to examine the first question, the social workers were asked a series of questions with regard to their first appearance in a legislative committee. The findings indicated that when they first participated in a committee meeting, the social workers ranged in age from 35–71 years old (M = 40.38, SD = 7.87). They had been employed as social workers for 10 to 45 years (M = 16.47, SD 6.44). Almost half (48.5%) worked in a national government ministry, over a third (37%) in a nonprofit organization, and 14.5% in local government. The role distribution of the social workers in each sector is presented in Figure 1.

As can be seen, about four-fifths of the participants from all three sectors held supervisory (team head, supervisor) or executive (administrator) roles, while only about a fifth were line workers.

The second question pertained to psychological engagement in politics, which was measured by three variables: political interest, political efficacy, and partisanship. A one-way MANOVA performed to examine group differences in interest in national and local politics showed a significant difference: $F(2, 187) = 7.81$, $p < .001$, $\eta^2 = .08$. ANOVAs were then undertaken for

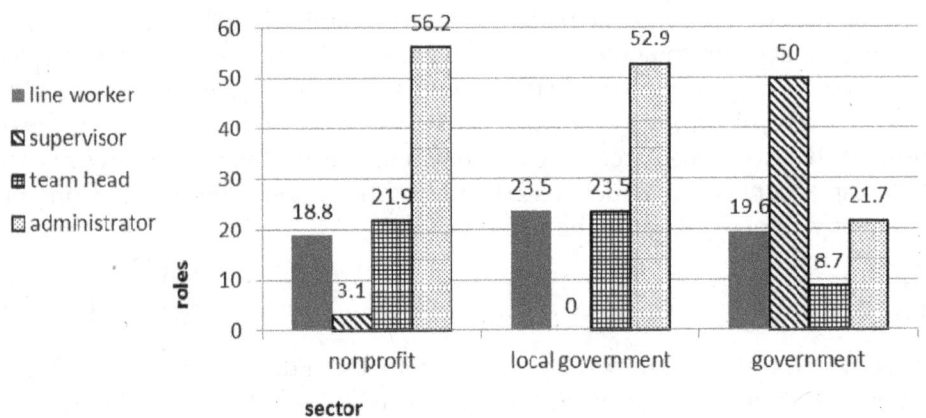

FIGURE 1 Social workers' role distribution by sector.

each policy level. A significant group difference was found only in interest in national politics ($F(2,187) = 15.24$, $p < .001$. $\eta^2 = .08$), with the study group showing greater interest ($M = 4.12$ $SD = .91$) than the comparison group ($M = 3.59$ $SD = .91$). The significant group difference at the national level remained when age and education were included in the equation (ANCOVAs). They also remained when a two-way MANOVA (2 groups × 3 organizational affiliations) was performed in order to examine whether the group difference in political interest stemmed from differences in organizational affiliation. However, the difference disappeared when seniority was included. In other words, the group difference in political interest was anchored in the difference in the seniority of the social workers in the two groups.

A one-way MANOVA performed to examine group differences in a sense of political efficacy showed no significant difference: $F(1, 188) = 2.42$, $p > .05$. On the whole, the social workers endorsed low to moderate political efficacy both on the local level (the study group: $M = 2.77$, $SD = 0.96$, the comparison group: $M = 2.78$, $SD = 0.88$) and on the national level (the study group: $M = 2.33$, $SD = 0.82$, the comparison group: $M = 2.14$, $SD = 0.87$).

A one-way ANOVA performed to examine group differences in partisanship showed no significant difference: $F(1, 188) = 0.10$, $p > .05$. On the whole, the social workers endorsed a moderate level of partisanship. In the study group, $M = 3.34$ ($SD = 1.2$). In the comparison group: $M = 3.28$ ($SD = 1.13$).

A one-way ANOVA performed to examine the third question, which related to differences in the two groups' policy practice training, yielded a significant difference: $F(4,185) = 14.67$, $p < .001$, $\eta^2 = .07$. The study group reported having received more policy practice training ($M = 3.01$, $SD = 1.28$) than the comparison group ($M = 2.34$, $SD = 1.14$). ANCOVAs controlling for group differences in seniority, education, and age similarly showed that the study group had received more policy practice training than the comparison group, implying that the groups' differences in policy practice training did not stem from group differences in seniority, education, and age. A two-way MANOVA (2 groups × 3 organizational affiliations) undertaken in order to examine whether the group difference in policy practice training stemmed from differences in organizational affiliation showed a significant difference, indicating that the group difference in training did not result from differences in organizational affiliation.

A one-way MANOVA was performed to examine the fourth question, with regard to group differences in engagement in policy practice at the organizational and governmental levels. The analysis showed a significant difference: $F(3, 186) = 16.28$, $p < .001$, $\eta^2 = .21$. Means, standard deviations, and the ANOVA results for each policy level are presented in Table 3.

As can be seen, the study group showed greater engagement in policy practice both on the organizational and national levels. ANCOVAs controlling

TABLE 3 Engagement in Policy Practice: Means, Standard Deviations and ANOVA ($N = 190$)

Involvement in policy practice at the:	The study group ($n = 95$)		The comparison group ($n = 95$)		Total ($N = 190$)	
	M	SD	M	SD	F (1,188)	η^2
Organizational level	4.09	1	3.35	1.17	16.53***	0.1
National level	3.21	1.32	2.08	1.17	60.25***	0.17

***$p < .001$.

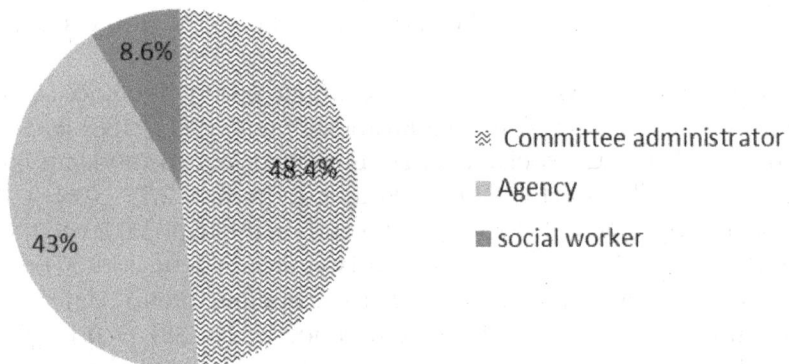

FIGURE 2 Distribution of initiation of the first appearance ($n = 95$).

for differences in seniority, education, or age similarly showed that the study group was more engaged in policy practice than the comparison group. A two-way MANOVA (2 groups × 3 organizational affiliations) conducted to examine whether the group difference in engagement in policy practice resulted from differences in organizational affiliation also showed a significant group difference, indicating that the difference in engagement did not stem from differences in organizational affiliation.

The last question related to the initiators of the social workers' participation in legislative committees meetings. Figure 2 shows the distribution of the initiators.

As can be seen, nearly half of the first appearances were responses to invitations by the committee administrator, either directly to the social worker or to the agency where he or she worked. Somewhat over two fifths of the first appearances were initiated by the agency and about a tenth by the social workers themselves. A similar distribution characterized the rest of the appearances, though a somewhat higher proportion of them were initiated by the committee administrators and a somewhat lower proportion by the agency.

Four chi square tests were conducted to determine whether the initiator differed in the three sectors. Findings showed a significant sectoral difference in the initiators of the first appearance ($\chi^2 = 9.88; p < .001$). The majority of the appearances from the government sector were initiated by the committee administrator (56%) and the remainder by the social worker's organization. In contrast, half of the appearances from the local government sector were initiated by the social worker's agency, 43% by the committee administrator, and 7% by the individual social worker. In the nonprofit sector, a similar proportion of the initiatives came from the committee administrator (41.7%) or the nonprofit agency (38.9%), and the remainder (20%) by the individual social worker. No significant sectoral differences were found in the sources of initiation of most of the appearances ($\chi^2 = 4.69; p > .005$); nor was any significant difference found in the role of the social workers who initiated their first appearance ($\chi^2 = 7.81; p > .005$) and those who initiated most of their other appearances ($\chi^2 = 9.41; p > .005$).

As stated in the Method section, the social workers who initiated their committee appearances were asked why they did so. Although the question was open and they could give multiple responses, most gave only one. A content analysis of their replies yielded four distinguishable reasons.

The first, given by seven respondents, was the desire to place their clients' social problems on the public agenda. They stated that their clients came from excluded populations whose voices were not heard in public discourse, and that they wanted both the public and the *Knesset* members to be aware of the problems and to act on them:

I wanted to make the public aware of a subject that is close to my heart, that I encounter every day at work and that I believe is important that they know about.(Social worker from the nonprofit sector, man, Jewish, 62 years old)

It was my way of raising public awareness of the difficulties and needs of parents of children with disabilities in the Arab sector. (Social worker from the nonprofit sector, woman, Arab, 36 years old)

I wanted to represent and give voice to my clients. (Social worker from the nonprofit sector, woman, Jewish, 68 years old)

The second reason, given by six social workers, was that they regarded participation in legislative committees as a routine part of their role or job.

It was an integral part of my role. (Social worker from the local sector, woman, Arab, 59 years old)

My job definition included policy promotion through raising issues in the relevant legislative committees. (Social worker from the nonprofit sector, woman, Jewish, 35 years old)

The social workers who offered this reason were evidently employed in positions that required them to participate in legislative committees and to engage in policy practice.

The third reason, given by four respondents, was to promote a policy with respect to a particular issue:

> *I wanted to promote a clause providing universal hospital nursing care. I only attended those discussions.* (Social worker from the governmental sector, woman, Jewish, 62 years old)

> *I initiated several appearances to speak about concrete problems of Ethiopian immigrants.* (Social worker from the local sector, woman, Jewish, 53 years old)

The fourth reason, given by three social workers, consisted of a variety of personal motives: One worker said that he *"had a lot of free time"* (Social worker from the governmental sector, man, Jewish, 71 years old). Another explained that he was motivated by a sense of personal responsibility: *"There were only a few social workers in the organization and I knew that if I didn't participate [in the legislative committee meeting], no one would"* (Social worker from the local sector, woman, Jewish, 60 years old).

DISCUSSION

The study findings showed that the social workers in the study group did not only engage in legislative advocacy but also reported a level of general involvement in policy practice (both on the organizational and national levels) that was greater than that of a comparison group of social workers. As such, the study findings afford us a unique opportunity to better understand factors related to social workers' involvement in policy practice by documenting the features of the members of this group and the circumstances of their involvement in the legislative arena.

Before discussing the key findings of the study, three main limitations should be explained. First, the analysis was based, in part, on self-reported responses of the study group members on the circumstances surrounding their first appearance in a legislative committee. Given the time that has lapsed since, this raises issues of recall. Second, the study methodology necessitated the construction of a comparison group with the same features of age, seniority, education, and organizational affiliation of the study group. However due to the unique features of the study group, this effort was only partially successful. Finally, some of the research tools employed here were constructed specifically for the current study and clearly require further validity and reliability processes.

With these limitations in mind, the findings of the study can be seen to shed new light on the engagement of social workers in job-related policy practice. In regard to the organizational affiliation at their first appearance in legislative committee meetings, the findings showed that almost half of the study group members were employed by central government, over a third were nonprofit employees, and a tenth worked for local government. This differs substantially from the overall distribution of social workers in Israel, which indicates that most are employed by local government (Bar-Zuri, 2004). The findings also revealed that almost half of the social workers participated in the meetings at the initiative of the committee administrators. However, it was also the workplace (be it government, nonprofit or local agencies) in which the social workers were employed that encouraged them to attend the committee meetings (46% in the government sector, 50% in the local government sector, and 39% in the nonprofit sector).

The PPE conceptual framework (Gal & Weiss-Gal, in press) can be useful in making sense of these findings. In the case of legislative advocacy in the Israeli parliament, the relative accessibility of legislative committees clearly affords social workers from different sectors an opportunity to participate in the policy process. The institutional context created by the norms of the specific policy juncture studied here legitimized participation of social workers in the policy process within legislative committees for social workers in all the three different sectors.

Legislative committee administrators tend routinely to invite civil servants to attend meetings relating to their domains of responsibility. Since Israeli legislation requires civil servants in the social welfare sphere to be filled by qualified social workers, the institutional norm to invite civil servants and the legislation create opportunities for government-employed social workers to participate in the policy formulation process. In other words, Israeli social workers in government have more opportunities to participate in the policy formulation process than do social workers in local government or nonprofits, and this explains the marked presence of government-employed social workers in the study group.

It appears that the accessible institutional context was the backdrop for an organizational environment that, in many cases, encouraged the policy practice of the social workers. However the accessibility of the policy process at this particular juncture or the legislation pertaining to social worker positions within government cannot offer a satisfactory explanation for the fact that it was the social welfare agencies, either government or nonprofit, or the individual social worker that often initiated participation in the legislative committee deliberations. Apparently, the participation of social workers in legislative committees also depended much upon the organizational culture of the agencies in which the social workers were employed.

Social workers in diverse agencies participated in policy practice because their immediate working environment and its leadership encouraged (or, at the very least, enabled) them to do so. This is clear from the findings, which identify local government and nonprofit agencies as a major source of the initiative to participate in the legislative committee deliberations. Put more simply, while opportunities existed for policy practice and institutional norms legitimized this type of engagement among social workers, the agencies themselves were a facilitating component that played a crucial role in the process that led to the legislative advocacy of the social workers.

Facilitation is also reflected in the finding that, in all the sectors, the majority of the social workers that participated in the legislative committees held administrative positions within their workplace. This confirms the assumption, based on findings of previous studies (Ezell, 1993, 1994), that senior administrative positions in agencies and government offices facilitate greater engagement in policy practice, in general, and in legislative advocacy, in particular. It can be assumed that social workers in these positions have greater access to the policy arena, are more willing to engage in policy practice, and indeed are often expected to play a role in the policy process.

The study assumed that motivational factors, the third component in the PPE framework, would also play a role in the engagement of individual social workers in the policy process in the legislative arena. The findings only partially confirmed the role of the motivational variables examined in the study. They did not offer support for the assumption, based on previous work on social workers' political participation, that factors such as political efficacy, political interest and partisanship, played an independent role in the policy practice of social workers in the legislative arena. This conclusion suggests that the motivational basis for job-based policy practice involvement and for social workers' political participation do not necessarily overlap and that the two should be considered to be distinctive types of policy-related behavior. Further research is required to determine whether different factors do indeed influence job-based policy practice and more general political participation, as suggested by this study.

The findings did underscore the role of two motivational factors—seniority and policy practice training. In comparison to social workers who had not been engaged in legislative advocacy, the study group participants reported having more training in policy practice. Moreover, when the members of the study group first participated in a legislative committee meeting they were characterized by considerable working experience. Reaffirming previous work showing the positive link between policy practice training and engagement in this type of practice (Anderson & Harris, 2005; Rocha, 2000; Tower & Hartnett, 2011; Weiss-Gal & Savaya, 2012), the findings of this study appear to confirm that a sense of efficacy (based on experience and training) plays a role in motivating social workers to engage in policy practice.

The place of the motivation component is also reflected in the quantitative findings. These underscored that, at least in a minority of cases, individual motivation can also play an important role in policy practice. Around 10% of the appearances were initiated by the social workers themselves. Describing their reasons for this, the social workers described an urge to place clients' social problems on the public agenda, a sense that this was an integral part of their role as social workers, and a desire to promote a policy in a particular issue. Clearly further study is required to better flesh out the role of motivational factors on policy practice. Among others, it would be useful to examine additional motivational variables such as policy practice skills and knowledge on policy processes (Ritter, 2013).

In conclusion, the findings of this study contribute to a more empirically based understanding of the factors related to the engagement of social workers in job-related policy practice. Moreover, it would appear that the findings concerning a group of social workers who engaged in job-related policy practice in the legislative arena offer support for the usefulness of the PPE framework. They underscore that it is the intersect between its three components—Opportunity, Facilitation, and Motivation—which created a context that encouraged the involvement of social workers in a specific form of policy practice. The study findings emphasize the opportunity and facilitation components of the framework over the motivational (at least, as measured in this study). It found that institutional norms and rules of the legislative arena and the readiness of a workplace to facilitate the involvement of social workers in the policy process contributed much to the engagement of the social workers, studied here, in job-related policy practice. A sense of self-efficacy, due to seniority and policy practice training, further enhanced the readiness of the participants to engage in this type of practice.

These conclusions have implications for theory, research, practice and education. On a theoretical level the study expands our knowledge of factors associated with social workers' involvement in policy practice. Additional research is needed in order to further empirically test the PPE framework and to follow up on the apparent differences between the factors that impact upon involvement in job-based policy practice and in voluntary political participation. On a practical level, the study findings focus our attention on the social workers' workplaces as a facilitating element that plays a crucial role in encouraging their engagement in policy practice. The corollary of this is that a major focus of efforts to increase policy practice on the part of social workers should be directed to creating environments within workplaces in the different sectors that do indeed facilitate this type of social work intervention.

Lastly, the findings reinforce the importance of policy training in encouraging policy involvement by social workers. Schools of social work should increase and consolidate policy practice training in order to increase social work involvement in policy practice. Based on our findings, we can assume that this training should relate to the diverse opportunity, facilitation, and motivational components of this type of practice. Social work students need to have a sense that they have the efficacy to engage in policy practice, to know that opportunities in the policy formulation process exist for them to do so, and that the workplace can be crucial in impeding or enhancing their policy practice involvement.

FUNDING

This research was supported by The Israel Science Foundation (grant No. 3/08).

REFERENCES

Abramovitz, M. (1998). Social work and social reform: An arena of struggle. *Social Work*, *43*(6), 512–526.

Anderson, D. K., & Harris, B. M. (2005). Teaching social welfare policy: A comparison of two pedagogical approaches. *Journal of Social Work Education*, *41*(3), 511–526.

Bar-Zuri, R. (2004). *Social workers in Israel—A survey of developments in the field in the years 1990–2002*. Jerusalem, Israel: Ministry of Industry, Commerce and Labor (Hebrew).

Cochran, G., & Davis, K. (2012). Social work and the Uniform Accident and Sickness Policy Provision Law: A pilot project. *Social Work*, *57*(1), 39–48.

Colby, I. C. (2008). Social welfare policy as a form of social justice. In I. C. Colby (Ed.), *Comprehensive handbook of social work and social welfare: Social policy and policy practice* (Vol. 4) (pp. 113–127). Hoboken, NJ: Wiley.

CSWE (Council on Social Work Education). (2010). Mission statement. Retrieved from www.cswe.org/albout.aspx

Cummins, L. K., Byers, K. V., & Pedrick, L. (2011). *Policy practice for social workers: New strategies for a new era* (updated edition). Boston, MA: Allyn & Bacon.

Ellis, R. A. (2008). Policy practice. In I. C. Colby (Ed.), *Comprehensive handbook of social work and social welfare: Social policy and policy practice* (Vol. 4) (pp.129–143). Hoboken, NJ: Wiley.

Ezell, M. (1991). Administrators as advocates. *Administration in Social Work*, *15*(4), 1–18.

Ezell, M. (1993). The political activity of social workers: A post-Reagan update. *Journal of Sociology and Social Welfare*, *20*, 81–97.

Ezell, M. (1994). Advocacy practice of social workers. *Families in Society*, *75*, 36–46.

Gal, J., & Weiss-Gal, I. (2011). Social policy formulation and the role of professionals: The involvement of social workers in parliamentary committees in Israel. *Health and Social Care in the Community*, *19*, 158–167.

Gal, J., & Weiss-Gal, I. (2015). The "why" and "how" of policy practice. *British Journal of Social Work, 45*(4), 1083–1101.

Greene, R., & Knee, R. (1996). Shaping the policy practice agenda of social work in the field of aging. *Social Work, 41*(5), 553–560.

Hamilton, D., & Fauri, D. (2001). Social workers' political participation: Strengthening the political confidence of social work students. *Journal of Social Work Education, 37*(2), 321–332.

Hartnett, H., Harding, S., & Scanlon, E. (2005). NASW chapters: Executive directors' perceptions of factors which impede and encourage active member participation. *Journal of Community Practice, 13*(4), 69–83.

Hoefer, R. (2012). *Advocacy practice for social justice* (2nd ed.). Chicago, IL: Lyceum.

Hoefer, R. (2013). Social workers affecting social policy in the United States. In J. Gal & I. Weiss-Gal (Eds.), *Social workers affecting social policy: An international perspective on policy practice* (pp. 161–182). Bristol, UK: Policy Press.

Jacobson, W. B. (2001). Beyond therapy: Bringing social work back to human services reform contributors. *Social Work, 46*(1), 51–61.

Jansson, B. S. (2014). *Becoming an effective policy advocate: From policy practice to social justice* (7th ed.). Belmont, CA: Brooks/Cole.

Mendes, P. (2013). Social workers affecting social policy in Australia. In J. Gal & I. Weiss-Gal (Eds.), *Social workers affecting social policy: An international perspective* (pp. 17–38). Bristol, UK: Policy Press.

Mosley, J. (2013). Recognizing new opportunities: Reconceptualizing policy advocacy in everyday organizational practice. *Social Work, 58*(3), 231–239.

NASW (National Association of Social Workers). (2010). *Code of ethics*. Retrieved from www.socialworkers.org/pubs/code/code/asp.

Pierce, D. (1984). *Policy for the social work practitioner*. New York, NY: Longman.

Pierce, D. (2000). Policy practice. In J. Midgley, M. Tracy, & M. Livermore (Eds.), *The handbook of social policy* (pp. 53–63). Thousand Oaks, CA: Sage.

Ritter, J. A. (2007). Evaluating the political participation of licensed social workers in the new millennium. *Journal of Policy Practice, 6*(4), 61–78.

Ritter, J. A. (2008). A national study predicting social workers' levels of political participation: The role of resources, psychological engagement, and recruitment networks. *Social Work, 53*(4), 347–357.

Ritter, J. A. (2013). *Social work policy practice: Changing our community, nation, and the world*. Boston, MA: Pearson.

Rocha, C. J. (2000). Evaluating experiential teaching methods in a policy practice course: The case for service learning to increase political participation. *Journal of Social Work Education, 36*, 53–63.

Rocha, C., Poe, B., & Thomas, V. (2010). Political activities of social workers: Addressing perceived barriers to political participation. *Social Work, 55*(4), 317–325.

Rubinstein, A., & Medina, B. (2005). *Constitutional law in the State of Israel* (Vol. II). Tel-Aviv, Israel: Schocken Publishing House. (Hebrew).

Schneider, R., & Netting, E. (1999). Influencing social policy in a time of devolution: Upholding social work's great tradition. *Social Work, 44*(4), 349–357.

Teush, O. (2012). *The relationship between personal resources, psychological engagement in politics and recruitment networks, and the involvement of Israeli social workers in policy practice* (Unpublished master's thesis). Tel Aviv University, Israel. (Hebrew).

Tower, L. E., & Hartnett, H. P. (2011). An Internet-based assignment to teach students to engage in policy practice: A three-cohort study. *Journal of Policy Practice, 10*, 65–77.

Verba, S., Schlozman, K. L., & Brady, H. E. (1995). *Voice and equality: Civic voluntarism in American politics.* Cambridge, MA: Harvard University Press.

Weiss-Gal, I., & Gal, J. (2014). Social workers as policy actors. *Journal of Social policy, 43*(1), 19–36.

Weiss-Gal, I., & Levin, L. (2010). Social workers and policy-practice: An analysis of job descriptions in Israel. *Journal of Policy Practice, 9*, 183–200.

Weiss-Gal, I., & Savaya, R. (2012). A hands-on policy practice seminar for social workers in Israel: Description and evaluation. *Journal of Policy Practice, 11*(3), 139–157.

Zubrzycki, J., & McArthur, M. (2004). Preparing social work students for policy practice: An Australian example. *Social Work Education, 23*(4), 451–464.

Leaning Out: Exploring Organizational Advocacy Activities From an Open Systems Perspective

LAURI GOLDKIND

Graduate School of Social Service, Fordham University, New York, New York, USA

This article explores the effect of organizational culture on engagement with advocacy activities, both traditional and electronic. The Competing Values Framework offers a model for understanding how organizations' culture influences behavior. Using a sample of nonprofit providers from across the country, the author hypothesized that organizations that use electronic advocacy tools are more involved with advocacy activities of all types. A paper and pencil survey was used to collect data on organizational culture, advocacy tools and techniques, perceived effectiveness of the advocacy tools, policy goals, organizational sustainability goals as well as barriers and facilitators of electronic advocacy. The study used path modeling to describe the connections between organizational culture and engagement in advocacy activities. The article examines the barriers and facilitators of electronic advocacy, the penetration of electronic advocacy use in this sample of agencies and the perceptions of effectiveness associated with using these strategies; lastly, the implications of these findings for managers and organizational leaders are discussed.

The relationship between organizational culture, an organization's advocacy practice, and the adoption of innovation has been relatively unexplored by social scientists. Although each of these areas has been studied, the interaction of the three is still uncharted. Now more than ever, in a climate of scarce resources and intense competition, the ability of organizations to orient themselves to their external environments, navigate changing political and economic landscapes, and adapt relevant new technologies is critical. So, also, is an organization's ability to advocate effectively on behalf of its constituents.

The nonprofit sector has been growing steadily, both in size and financial impact, for more than a decade. Between 2001 and 2011, the number of nonprofits increased 25%, from 1,259,764 to 1,574,674. Impressively, the growth rate of the nonprofit sector has surpassed the rate of growth in both the business and government sectors (Roeger, Blackwood, & Pettijohn, 2012). Given the sector's significant growth, especially in a stagnant economy, as well as its prospects for further expansion, it is critical that we begin to understand the relationship between organizational culture, adaption to innovations, and advocacy, so that agency leaders are better informed as they attempt to grow their organizations and retain their ability to serve their constituents.

Study Purpose

Using the Competing Values Framework (CVF) as its theoretical orientation, this study examines the relationship between an organization's open systems focus, its internal structures, and its engagement in electronic advocacy activities. It asks the questions: Do organizations operating from an open systems perspective attend to their environments in ways that are significantly different from their more internally focused counterparts? Does this differential attention translate into higher rates of electronic advocacy behavior? In this case, the environment orientation, consistent with the CVF, is conceptualized as the forces external to the organization, to which the organization has limited to no control over but are central to an organization's success. Elements of the external environment might include the sociopolitical climate, the geographic region or community where an organization is situated as well as the changing demographics of an organization's clientele. The hypothesis this study specifically tests are:

- H1: Organizational "imperatives"—policy goals and organizational sustainability—are expected to have direct effects on organizational climate, electronic barriers and facilitators, the use of electronic advocacy strategies and, ultimately, upon the perceived effectiveness of those strategies.
- H2: Organizational climate is hypothesized to have direct effects on electronic advocacy barriers and facilitators, the use of electronic strategies and the perceived effectiveness of the use of these strategies.

H3: Electronic barriers and facilitators will have direct effects on the use of electronic advocacy strategies and organizations' perceptions of their effectiveness.

H4: The use of electronic advocacy strategies will have a direct effect on organizations' perceptions of their effectiveness.

LITERATURE REVIEW

About 34% of all nonprofit organizations are providers of direct human services. Such organizations are commonly referred to as human service organizations (HSOs) (Blackwood, 2012) and provide services such as case management, poverty relief, crisis intervention, workforce readiness, mental health, and child and family services. Delivering such services is a challenge: HSOs face ever-increasing pressure to monetize and quantify their service delivery models and outcomes to funders and other external constituents while engaging clients who face difficulties rooted in challenges on the interpersonal, community, and/or structural levels.

Given the intense pressure on HSOs to do more with less, to provide unduplicated services, and to uphold their missions that often include client empowerment, advocacy should be integral to the operations of this sector (Smith & Pekkanen, 2012). However, organizational advocacy in support of policy change and sustainability is not a common feature of the behaviors of such organizations (Almog-Bar & Schmid, 2013).

Nonprofit Advocacy

Advocating for disenfranchised groups, empowering constituents, and working on behalf of social justice frequently are considered central tenets of the human services sector (Berry, 2005; Mosley, 2011; Schachter, 2011). However, the level of policy advocacy engagement by nonprofit human service providers has been found to be relatively modest (Almog-Bar & Schmid, 2013; Kimberlin, 2010; Macindoe & Whalen, 2013). Many factors, including limited resources and knowledge and fear of reprisal from funders, contributes to the less than robust advocacy activities of this sector.

Electronic, Internet-based interactive tools (social media and the like) are facilitating the ways in which individuals and organizations engage in advocacy campaigns (Guo & Saxton, 2014; Nah & Saxton, 2013). Although there is some discussion in the literature about the types and goals of various advocacy activities undertaken by HSOs, there is general agreement that the nonprofit human services sector has a responsibility to uphold a civil society through advocacy activities and a belief that the human service sector is uniquely positioned to engage in these activities. Still, there is much to be understood about how and under what conditions agencies adopt the use of electronic advocacy tools.

Facilitators of Advocacy Practice

The growth and maintenance of an organizational advocacy program and the ability to meet advocacy objectives require organizational structures and supports. Facilitators of organizational advocacy include coalition membership, leadership support (including board support), and resources (Donaldson, 2007). Not surprisingly, organizations with greater capacity in terms of staff, dollars, and volunteers are more likely to engage in advocacy behaviors than organizations with fewer resources (Berry & Arons, 2003; Suarez, 2009). Gibelman and Kraft (1996) identify the type of agency, agency size, mission, functions, and staff expertise that are associated with the nature of an agency's advocacy practice. They also lay out a conceptual model of agency-level advocacy practice that elevates advocacy activities to the same status as agency's programmatic activities, and suggest that without resources (e.g., money, staff expertise, and technology), a robust agency advocacy agenda cannot be executed.

Organizational leadership may be one of the key factors that influences an agency's advocacy activities. De Vita, Montilla, Reid, and Fatiregun, (2004), Gibelman and Kraft (1996), Saidel and Harlan (1998), and Salamon (1995) all suggest that leadership and the leader's orientation, vision, and commitment to advocacy are critical factors in an organization's advocacy engagement.

Barriers to Advocacy Practice

As agencies are pressured to demonstrate effectiveness and efficiency with ever-shrinking resources, advocacy, and civic engagement activities are often considered nonessential. Time, resources, and expertise are the most frequently mentioned barriers to advocacy activities (Donaldson, 2007; McNutt & Boland, 1999). Given that advocacy should be a singular feature of the sector, it is noteworthy that a significant number of organizational leaders do not think they are competent to engage in these activities.

In terms of the use of electronic advocacy specifically, these same barriers seem to exist (McNutt & Boland, 1999). However, McNutt (2008) goes further, and suggests that similar to the Digital Divide discussed in the early 2000s, an emergent Organizational Digital Divide threatens to leave small, less-capitalized organizations behind because they lack both the access to technology tools and the human capital to deploy them.

E-advocacy Tools and Tactics

Media tools (Twitter, Facebook, text messaging, etc.) are revolutionizing policy advocacy practices in the United States and around the world. Fitzgerald and McNutt (1997, p. 3) define electronic advocacy as "the use of technologically intensive media as a means to influence stakeholders to effect policy change." Increasingly pervasive, these strategies and tools cannot be ignored by nonprofit leaders wishing to remain relevant in their increasingly competitive climates.

"Social media" and "Web 2.0" are terms used to describe technologies that support interaction and networking, user-generated content, and the pooling of collective intelligence (Bryant, 2006; Germany 2006; Kanter & Fine, 2010; O'Reilly 2005). These tools tend to be interactive rather than unidirectional; users are connected to each other and create feedback loops or information channels between actors rather than transmitting information in a single direction (historically, from an organization to a constituent/stakeholder). These technologies tend to be cloud applications where the Internet is used as the platform.

Social network sites are one of the fastest growing technological arenas. They have become an important advocacy tool, regularly used by political campaigns, advocacy groups, and social movements. Such sites function as virtual hubs on the Internet, allowing individuals, organizations, and institutions to connect with one another. Social networking sites such as Facebook, MySpace, LinkedIn, Google +, and others are driven by user participation and user-generated content (Tredinnick, 2006). Through interactions with stakeholders such as clients, donors, and volunteers on such sites, organizations seek to develop relationships with important publics.

Organizational Culture and the Competing Values Framework

Schein (1983), a leading scholar of organizational culture, defines it as:

> the pattern of basic assumptions which a given group has invented, discovered, or developed in learning to cope with its problems of external adaptation and internal integration, which have worked well enough to be considered valid, and, therefore, to be taught to new members as the correct way to perceive, think, and feel in relation to those problems. (p. 186)

Since 1980, more than 4,600 articles have examined organizational culture (Hartnell, Ou, & Kinicki, 2011). Organizational scholars agree that culture has a powerful influence on an organization's success and effectiveness (Cameron & Quinn, 2011; Greenhalgh, MacFarlane, & Peacock, 2009; Khazanchi, Lewis, & Boyer, 2007; Schein, 2006), and organizational culture is the driver of effectiveness, innovation, staff satisfaction, and a broad range of other organizational characteristics.

One theoretical perspective for understanding organizational culture is the Competing Values Framework (CVF). CVF organizes the tensions, contradictions, and opportunities that organizational leaders encounter across four broad quadrants. It is widely used in the literature and as an assessment has been administered to more than 10,000 organizations globally (Cameron, Quinn, DeGraff, & Thakor, 2006; Ostroff, Kinicki, & Tamkins, 2003).

The CVF offers one meta-theoretical model that is inclusive of the values that underlie organizational climates (Gifford, Zammuto, & Goodman, 2002; Quinn & McGrath, 1985; Quinn & Rohrbaugh, 1983). It calls attention to "how opposing values exist in organizations" and how "individual organizations are likely to embrace different mixtures of values that are reflected in their desired ends and in the means to attain them, such as their structural designs and mechanisms of co-ordination and control" (Zammuto & O'Connor, 1992, p. 711).

The CVF proposes that organizational effectiveness criteria can best be understood when organized along two fundamental dimensions—flexibility versus control and internal versus external orientation. Depicted as a four-quadrant model, the horizontal axis represents organizational focus as either internal or external; the vertical axis focuses on organizational adaptability as either flexible or controlled (Zafft & Adams, 2008).

The two axes split the framework into four competing quadrants (also known as profiles). The quadrants are the Human Relations model (flexible structure with an internal focus), the Open Systems model (flexible structure and external focus), the Internal Process model (controlled structure and internal focus), and the Rational Goal model (controlled structure and external focus; Lawrence, Lenk, & Quinn, 2009; Quinn, 1988). Each quadrant of the model has a competing opposite; for example, the Human Relations quadrant, which emphasizes a flexible structure with an internal focus, is diametrically opposed to the Rational Goal model with its focus on a controlled structure and external focus.

This study explores the effect of organizational culture, and specifically an Open System's orientation, on the adoption of electronic advocacy strategies. Organizations operating in the Open Systems quadrant of the CVF focus on an adaptation to the external environment and have flexible structures. Leaders in these organizations value and support strategies that foster growth, innovation, and creativity (Kalliath, Bluedorn, & Gillespie, 1999).

Thus, the Open Systems model emphasizes readiness for change and innovation, and norms and values are associated with growth, resource acquisition, creativity, and adaptation. Climate dimensions associated with this orientation are (a) flexibility and innovation—an orientation toward change (e.g., Garrahan & Stewart, 1992; King & Anderson, 1995) as well as the extent of encouragement and support for new ideas and innovative approaches (e.g., West & Farr, 1990); (b) an outward focus—the extent to which the organization is responsive to the needs of the customer and the marketplace in general (Kiesler & Sproull, 1982; West & Farr, 1990); and (c) reflexivity—a concern with reviewing and reflecting upon objectives, strategies, and work processes, in order to adapt to the wider environment (West, 1996, 2000).

Since electronic advocacy tools and tactics are new and innovative and foster growth within an organization, this study hypothesizes that organizations operating most strongly in the Open Systems quadrant will make greater use not only of traditional advocacy strategies but of electronic advocacy tools and tactics than other organizations.

METHOD

Design

The study used a mailed survey to reach a national sample of human services executives. Cover letters and paper survey instruments were mailed to more than 3,800 executive directors of human service agencies. The letter to agency executives invited them to participate in a study exploring how agencies engage in policy advocacy work and use electronic media tools in particular. It also introduced the principal investigator as a faculty member with a personal interest in the subject matter of the study, and laid out the study's objectives. Following this initial mailing, four follow-up reminder postcards were sent in an attempt to increase the response rate.

Anonymous surveys were returned in postage-paid envelopes; agency leaders did not submit their names or the names of their organizations. This research was conducted with Institutional Review Board approval from the authors' university.

Study Sample

The executive directors of all Category P20 human services providers with budgets greater than \$30,000 per year ($N = 3,804$), as identified by the National Taxonomy of Exempt Entities (NTEE), were included in the sample. The NTEE system is used by the IRS and the National Center for Charitable Statistics (NCCS) to classify nonprofit organizations (Sumariwalla, 1986); Category P20 identifies human service providers.

Two hundred sixty-four completed surveys were returned. Despite using tactics to increase the response rate suggested by Dillman (2000) and others, such as sending four rounds of reminder postcards and offering a post-survey incentive, the response rate was 7%. It should be noted, however, that organizational researchers (e.g., Hager, Wilson, Pollak, & Rooney, 2003) suggest that surveys of organizations frequently report noticeably lower return rates than do surveys of individuals.

Instruments

To capture Quinn and Rohrbaugh's (1981) CVF, parts of Patterson et al.'s (2005) Organizational Climate Measure were used. The Child Welfare

Electronic Advocacy Survey, developed by McNutt (2007), was used to capture the barriers and facilitators of advocacy activity.

Organizational climate. Three subscales of the Organizational Climate Measure (Patterson et al., 2005) were used to capture the organization's place in the Open System's quadrant of the CVF: Outward Focus composed of five questions; Innovation and Flexibility composed of six items; and Reflexivity composed of five questions. Table 1 identifies the exact items that were used.

Sixteen Likert-type items comprised the three subscales of flexibility, outward focus, and reflexivity that were used by the respondents to indicate the degree to which they believed that their organization behaved in the Open Systems Model of the CVF. More specifically, the respondents indicated whether the attribute in question was *Definitely false* (1), *Mostly false* (2), *Mostly true* (3) and *Definitely true* (4) of their organization.

An initial confirmatory factor analysis on these 16 items indicated that the Patterson et al. (2005) factor structure provided a suboptimal fit to these

TABLE 1 Organizational Climate Measure Items

Subscale	Item
Outward Focus	This organization is quite inward looking; it does not concern itself with what is happening in the marketplace.
	Ways of improving service to the customer are not given much thought.
	Customer needs are not considered top priority here.
	This company is slow to respond to the needs of the customer.
	This organization is continually looking for new opportunities in the marketplace.
Innovation & Flexibility	New ideas are readily accepted here.
	This company is quick to respond when changes need to be made.
	People in this organization are always searching for new ways of looking at problems.
	Assistance in developing new ideas is readily available.
	This organization is very flexible; it can quickly change procedures to meet new conditions and solve problems as they arise.
	Management here is quick to spot the need to do things differently.
Reflexivity	In this organization, the way people work together is changed readily in order to improve performance.
	There are regular discussions as to whether people in the organization are working effectively together.
	The methods used by this organization to get the job done are often discussed.
	In this organization, time is taken to review organizational objectives.
	In this organization, objectives are modified in light of changing circumstances.

TABLE 2 Organizational Climate Factor Structure and Factor Intercorrelations

Variable	Innovation - Flexibility	Outward Focus	Reflexivity
New ideas accepted	.65*		
Organization responsive to changes	.69*		
Management quick to identify needs	.57*		
Org is flexible	.80*		
Assistance for new ideas	.65*		
People look for new ways to think about problems	.65*		
Organization looks for new opportunities in the environment	.50*		
Organization is inward looking		.49*	
Service improvement not a priority		.86*	
Client needs not priority		.80*	
Organization slow to respond to clients		.67*	
Staff reconfigured to improve performance			.63*
Service delivery discussed			.67*
Review of team effectiveness			.72*
Objectives modified			.60*
Reviews organization goals			.61*
Inter-factor Correlations	**Innovation - Flexibility**	**Outward Focus**	**Reflexivity**
Innovation-Flexibility	—	—	—
Outward Focus	.41*	—	—
Reflexivity	.75*	.37*	—

*$p < .05$.

data ($\chi^2 = 280.13$ (101), $p < .001$, CFI = .88, RMSEA = .08). However, one item failed to load on the factor to which it was assigned by Patterson et al. (2005). Given these findings, the confirmatory factor model was re-specified, moving this item from the Outward Focus factor to which it was initially assigned to the Innovation/Flexibility factor.

The re-specified model provided an improved and now satisfactory fit to the data ($\chi^2 = 230.84$ (101), $p < .001$, CFI = .91, RMSEA = .07). Essentially, the revised factor structure replicates the original Patterson et al. (2005) factors structure with sole exception of this one item (see Table 2). Moreover, each of the loadings of three scales that operationally define organizational culture is substantial and statistically significant. The internal consistency reliability coefficients for the three factors are Innovation/Flexibility ($\alpha = .84$), Outward Focus ($\alpha = .78$) and Reflexivity ($\alpha = .78$).

Barriers and facilitators of electronic advocacy use. Eleven items asked the respondents to characterize the degree to which various structural characteristics of the organization serve as barriers to, or facilitators of, the use of electronic strategies for advocacy. They were adapted from the Child Welfare Study mentioned previously (McNutt, 2007). For example, "structural characteristics" included board support, financial support, technology infrastructure, and senior leadership support, among others.

The response scale for the 11 items referencing these characteristics ranged from −5 through 0 to +5, where −5 indicated that the characteristic was the greatest possible barrier to advocacy activities and +5 indicated that the resource functioned as the greatest possible facilitator of those same advocacy activities. These 11 items were summed to form a unidimensional scale, and had an internal consistency reliability coefficient of $\alpha = .85$.

Engagement in advocacy activities. Engagement in advocacy activities and the exploration of the use of electronic Internet-based strategies were captured using an adapted version of McNutt's Child Welfare Advocacy Survey. The organizations who participated in the study were asked to describe their level of use of an array of 27 electronic advocacy strategies, including social media tools, for example, Facebook, blogs, and podcasting, as well as direct electronic communication tools such as e-mail, chat rooms, and Listservs. Specifically, the participants were asked to indicate whether they used each strategy (1) *not at all*; (2) *sometimes*; or (3) *regularly*. For the purposes of operationalizing the use of electronic advocacy strategies, a unidimensional summary score, (i.e., the mean of the electronic strategy items) was estimated for each of the organizations in the study sample. The internal consistency reliability of this summary measure is $\alpha s = .90$.

Data Analysis

As noted previously, a confirmatory factor analysis was first used to test the factor structure of the items developed by Patterson et al. (2005). Once this was completed and the data structure was finalized, the analytic focus of this investigation turned to the development of a path analytic model that explains traditional and electronic advocacy use by human service organizations. This path model is developed to explain the relationships—direct and indirect—between aspects of organizational culture and the use of electronic and traditional advocacy strategies.

RESULTS

The tenure of the 264 participating organizations ranged from 4 to 155 years old, with a mean of 36 years and a median of 25 years. On average, the organizations' budgets were $500,000, but ranged from less than $50,000 (9%) to more than $5,000,000 (27%). Sixty-three percent of respondents reported having an individual who is responsible for coordinating technology on their staff. In addition, 66% reported having memberships in coalitions or other affinity group organizations. A substantial majority of the respondents (87%)

report spending 25% or less of their organization's time engaged in advocacy activities.

The univariate descriptive statistics for the 16 items and each of the three organizational culture measures on which they are based are reported in Table 3. As shown, the respondents generally characterized their organizations as sensitive to the nuances of the external environment. That is to say, the means of the 16 items, as well as the three organizational culture measures they comprise, indicate that, on average, the 16 attributes were seen as *mostly true* ($\bar{x} > 3$) of the organizations in the study sample. Stated somewhat differently, and using the parlance of the CVF, these are, on average, "outwardly focused" organizations.

Barriers and Facilitators of Electronic Advocacy Use

The survey instrument includes 11 items that asked the respondents to characterize the degree to which various structural characteristics of the organization functioned as either a barrier to, or as a facilitator of, the use of electronic advocacy strategies. "Structural" characteristics include board support, financial support, technology infrastructure, and senior leadership support, among others. Specifically, the respondents rated each organizational resource on a scale from −5 (*greatest barrier*) to +5 (*greatest facilitator*). As seen in Table 4, with the exception of Resistance to Technological Change, all of the means are positively signed, indicating that these structural characteristics are generally seen as facilitators, not barriers, to electronic advocacy strategy use, albeit to different degrees. More specifically, Senior Executive Support ($M = 2.88$), Board Support ($M = 2.37$), Coalition Membership ($M = 2.19$) and Expertise ($M = 2.08$) were viewed as the structural resources most supportive of electronic advocacy use. Excepting Resistance to Technological Change, the remaining structural characteristics in Table 4, were also viewed as facilitators of electronic advocacy use but to lesser degrees (all means < 1.50).

The descriptive statistics for the electronic strategy variables are presented in Table 5. Note that the percentage of the organizational sample using each strategy at least sometimes is reported as the mean proportion, that is, the percentage of respondents who reported using that strategy (see the column labeled $\bar{x}$). As seen in this table, the most widely used electronic strategies were e-mails to decision makers (56%) and e-mails used internally to coordinate policy advocacy efforts (52%).

With respect to the social media advocacy strategies, the most prevalent strategy was the use of social networking (49%), for example, LinkedIn and Facebook. All of the remaining social media advocacy strategies were much less utilized (< 15% of the agencies used these *sometimes* or *more frequently*). Finally, with regard to "other" electronic strategies, the most widely used of these strategies were online fundraising (30%) and instant messaging

TABLE 3 Organizational Culture Measures

Item	n	$\bar{x}$	SD
Innovation/Flexibility	**262**	**3.17**	**0.48**
New ideas are readily accepted here.	262	3.34	0.62
This organization is quick to respond when changes need to be made.	261	3.19	0.62
Management here is quick to spot the need to do things differently.	259	3.23	0.62
This organization is very flexible; it can quickly change procedures to meet new conditions and solve problems as they arise.	260	3.19	0.71
Assistance in developing new ideas is readily available.	258	2.95	0.72
People in this organization are always searching for new ways of looking at problems.	257	3.08	0.71
This organization is continually looking for new opportunities in the environment.	259	3.24	0.70
Outward Focus	**260**	**3.60**	**0.49**
Organization is not inward looking.	257	3.32	0.75
Service improvement is a priority.	259	3.64	0.62
Clients are a priority.	261	3.78	0.57
Organization is not slow to respond to clients.	261	3.67	0.58
Reflexivity	**261**	**3.11**	**0.49**
In this organization, the way people work together is readily change in order to improve performance.	255	2.97	0.65
The methods used by this organization to get the job done are often discussed.	259	3.21	0.66
There are regular discussions as to whether people in the organization are working together effectively.	260	3.02	0.72
In this organization, objectives are modified in light of changing circumstances.	256	3.15	0.64
In this organization, time is taken to review organizational goals and objectives.	259	3.23	0.69

(30%), followed by online volunteer recruiting (26%), online mapping (22%), and secure intranet for internal communications (22%).

Understanding Electronic Advocacy Use

Figure 1 presents the "trimmed" path diagram for the estimated structural equation model. Initially, this model was estimated as a fully recursive model, i.e., all possible unidirectional paths moving from left to right in the diagram were estimated. Subsequently, any statistically insignificant path

TABLE 4 Barriers and Facilitators of Electronic Advocacy

	n	$\bar{x}$	SD
Board Support	250	2.37	2.31
Fiscal Support	250	1.32	2.86
Technology Infrastructure	247	1.20	2.48
Senior Executive support	250	2.88	2.16
Technology Champions	243	0.99	2.52
Coalition Membership	243	2.08	2.22
Advocacy Core Activity	248	1.36	2.73
Universal Access	232	0.84	2.44
Space	245	0.72	2.53
Resistance	236	0.07	2.03
Expertise	247	2.00	2.52

($p > .05$) was removed from the model. As a result, this diagram includes only the statistically significant (standardized) direct effects of each variable on those variables hypothesized to be affected by it. These direct effects represent only part of the (standardized) total effect of each variable in the model. In fact, the total effect of each variable in the model can be decomposed into its direct effect plus its indirect effect(s) on variables that appear subsequent to it in Figure 1.

As seen in Figure 1, the "imperatives" of human service organizations, i.e., their policy goals and their system maintenance activities (organizational sustainability), are considered to be determinants of the type of organizational culture that evolves to service these imperatives. Consistent with the tenets of Open Systems Theory, human service organizations with a greater emphasis on "system maintenance" activities, i.e., increasing their visibility, capacity, access to volunteers and resources, adopt a more externally focused organizational culture (Organizational Sustainability, $\beta = .36, p < .05$). On the other hand, and contrary to expectation, these organizations' policy goals do not have a direct effect on the type of organizational culture that develops. That is to say, human service organizations with a greater commitment to a constituent-driven advocacy agenda do not adopt a more externally focused organizational culture.

Again, consistent with expectation, Policy Goals ($\beta = .27, p < .05$) and Organizational Climate ($\beta = .41, p < .05$) have significant direct effects on Electronic Advocacy Barriers and Facilitators, one of the two key "infrastructure" variables in the model. Organizational Sustainability has no such direct effect; however, it does have a substantial indirect effect on Electronic Advocacy Barriers and Facilitators via its effect on Organizational Climate (indirect effect (i.e.) $= .15, p < .05$). Stated somewhat differently, "systems maintenance activities" do have an effect on this infrastructure component but that effect is entirely mediated by Organizational Climate (Patterson et al., 2005).

TABLE 5 Electronic Advocacy Tools and Techniques

Strategy Type	$\bar{x}$	N
Electronic Advocacy Strategies		
E-mail to Coordinate Policy Influence Efforts within organization	.52	258
E-mail to Coordinate Policy Influence Efforts outside of organization	.43	258
Electronic Mail Discussion List About Policy Issues (List serve)	.27	256
Electronic Mail [E-Mail] to Decision Makers	.56	259
Newsgroups	.16	258
Distribution Lists [Mass E-Mail Distribution]	.45	258
Chat Rooms	.00	257
Social Media Advocacy Strategies		
Blogs	.11	258
RSS Feeds (Really Simple Syndication)	.03	252
Wikis (Wikipedia)	.07	257
Photo Sharing (Picassa, Flicker)	.11	255
Podcasting	.02	255
Video Sharing (YouTube)	.14	259
Micro blogging (Twitter)	.15	257
Social Networking (LinkedIn, Facebook, etc)	.49	259
Social Bookmarking (Delicious, Digg, StumbleUpon, etc)	.01	255
Other Electronic Strategies		
Online Fundraising (secure donation sites or shop for a cause sites)	.30	259
Video-Teleconferencing	.12	259
Online Survey Research	.19	259
Online Volunteer Recruiting	.26	260
Online Mapping (Like Google Earth or Google Maps)	.22	257
Secure Intranet for Coordinating Activities private communication	.22	259
Meet ups [a tool that helps to organize face-to-face meetings]	.09	256
Instant Messaging, Texting, and Short Message Systems	.30	260
Virtual Reality Simulation [Like Second Life]	.08	256
OnLine Petitions	.04	257
Web-based Conferencing	.17	260

With respect to the second key infrastructure variable, the use of Electronic Advocacy Strategies, Policy Goals has a statistically significant direct effect on this variable ($\beta = .28, p < .05$) as well as a significant indirect effect via its impact on Electronic Advocacy Barriers and Facilitators (i.e., = .06, $p < .05$). Organizational Sustainability also has a significant direct effect on this infrastructure variable ($\beta = .30, p < .05$) as well as a significant compound indirect effect via Organizational Climate and Electronic Advocacy Barriers and Facilitators (i.e. = .03, $p < .05$). Organizational Climate's effect on the use of Electronic Advocacy Strategies is also substantial and completely mediated via its effect on Electronic Advocacy Barriers and Facilitators (i.e. = .09, $p < .05$). Not surprisingly, the latter variable, Electronic Advocacy

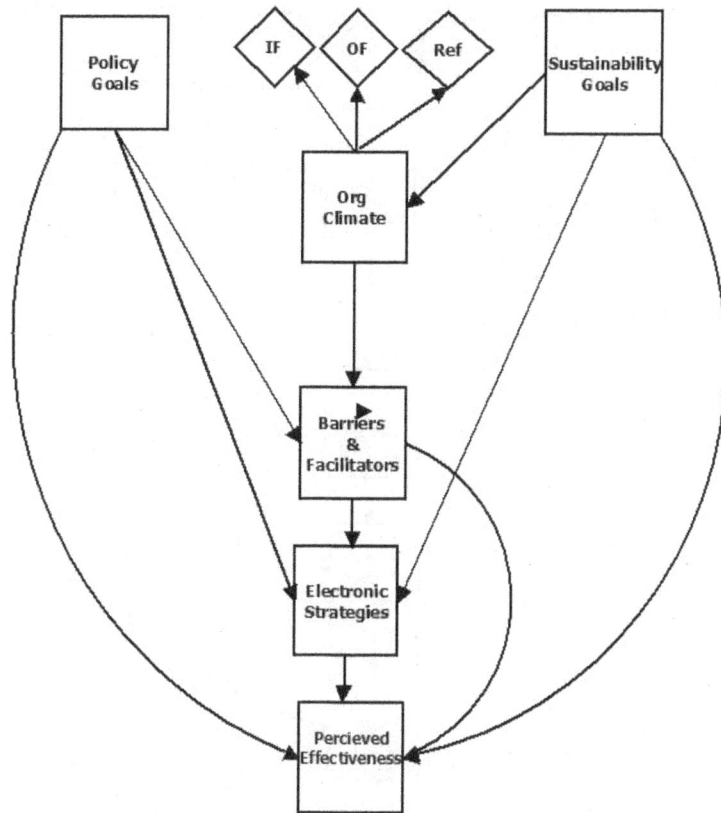

FIGURE 1 Conceptual model.

Barriers and Facilitators has a significant direct effect on the use of Electronic Advocacy Strategies ($\beta = .23, p < .05$).

As can be seen in Figure 2, the ultimate outcome of the model, the Perceived Effectiveness of Using Electronic Advocacy Strategies, Policy Goals ($\beta = .23, p < .05$), Organizational Sustainability ($\beta = .23, p < .05$), Electronic Advocacy Barriers and Facilitators ($\beta = .21, p < .05$) and the Use of Electronic Advocacy Strategies ($\beta = .21, p < .05$) each have significant direct effects on Perceived Effectiveness. The first three of these variables also have a number of statistically significant indirect effects. Specifically, Policy Goals has a significant indirect effect via Electronic Advocacy Barriers and Facilitators (i.e. = .06, $p < .05$) and the Use of Electronic Strategies (i.e. = .06, $p < .05$). It also has a significant compound indirect effect on Perceived Effectiveness via its effect on Electronic Advocacy Barriers and Facilitators and through this variable on the Use of Electronic Advocacy Strategies which, in turn, has an effect on Perceived Effectiveness (i.e. = .01, $p < .05$).

Organizational Sustainability has a significant indirect effect on Perceived Effectiveness via the Use of Electronic Advocacy Strategies (i.e.

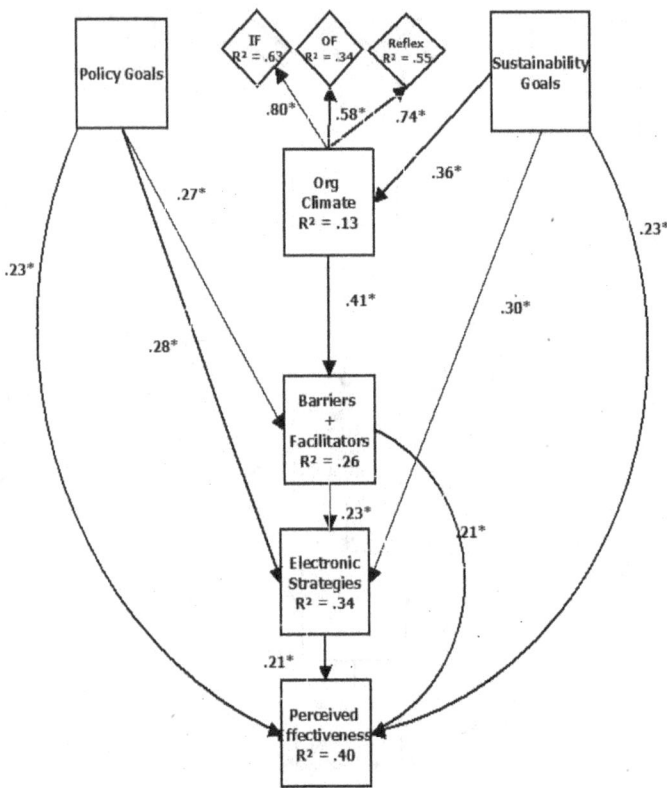

FIGURE 2 Path model.

= .06, p < .05). It also has a statistically significant compound indirect effect which includes Organizational Climate and Electronic Advocacy Barriers and Facilitators as mediators (i.e. = .03, $p < .05$). There is also a marginally significant, second compound indirect effect which includes three intervening variables, i.e., Organizational Climate, Electronic Advocacy Barriers and Facilitators as well as the Use of Electronic Advocacy Strategies (i.e. = .01, $p = .07$).

Organizational Climate's effect on Perceived Effectiveness is entirely indirect or mediated. It has a sizeable and statistically significant indirect effect on Perceived Effectiveness via its impact on Electronic Barriers and Facilitators (i.e. = .08, $p < .05$). In addition, it has a significant, compound indirect effect on Perceived Effectiveness via two intervening variables, i.e., Electronic Advocacy Barriers and Facilitators and the Use of Electronic Advocacy Strategies (i.e. = .02, $p < .05$). Lastly, Electronic Advocacy Barriers and Facilitators exerts part of its impact on Perceived Effectiveness indirectly via its effect on the Use of Electronic Advocacy Strategies (i.e. = .05, $p = .05$)

DISCUSSION

Two of the greatest challenges facing HSOs are to better service their advocacy agendas and to ensure their ongoing ability to do so. By capitalizing on the new, digital media, which are designed for this very purpose—it would seem that both objectives can be achieved. However, very little data, for or against this assertion, exists. This effort begins to address this deficit. Specifically, we propose and test a model that links the aforementioned organizational imperatives—policy goal achievement and organizational sustainability—to the development of a particular organizational "culture" that is designed to promote these ends. Drawing upon Open Systems Theory, the author has demonstrated that human service organizations' sustainability, but surprisingly not their policy agendas, are important determinants of the "organizational cultures" that evolve to service these two organizational imperatives. As such, the "systems maintenance activities" of human service organizations—achieving greater organizational visibility, capacity, access to volunteers and acquisition of resources—are indirectly serviced by the development of an "externally focused" organizational culture which facilitates the adoption of newer digital "tools" the effectiveness of which these organizations attest to. While servicing an advocacy agenda is not a determinant of this more "facilitative" organizational culture, it is nonetheless the case that the policy agendas of these organizations have significant direct impacts on the acquisition of these digital tools and the perception that they are effective in promoting those agendas. In effect, then, we find, admittedly qualified, support for the claim that new "digital age" tools like social media are instrumental in helping human service organizations realize their objectives. Our support is necessarily qualified because the "evidence" for this claim rests on the subjective assessments of the members of these organizations. Needed are more controlled comparisons between human service organizations that do, and do not, adopt these new digital technologies. Until that time, however, the data provided herein can be considered consistent with, but not proof of, the possible benefits of adopting these media to achieve essential organizational objectives.

Limitations

This study has several limitations that should be noted. First, as a matter of record, The National Taxonomy of Exempt Entities identifies ($N = 3,800$) general human service organizations with budgets of more than $30,000. Because this list of organizations is the most current and complete list of human service organizations available, it was selected to provide the sampling frame for this study. However, only 7% ($n = 262$) of these organizations participated in this study. Given that fact, it is reasonable to have some concerns about the representativeness of the sample and the generalizability of the findings.

In addition, with respect to the mediating variable in our model—organizational barriers and facilitators of electronic communication technologies—it might have been useful to have also directly inquired about the corresponding organizational barriers and facilitators associated with the use of traditional communication technologies. Unfortunately, space limitations in the survey instrument precluded doing so.

Finally, organizational surveys require someone to speak for the entire organization (Hager et al., 2003), and the question remains whether and to what extent any one individual can be said to be "fully sighted" about the broad array of issues of a survey such as the one used in this investigation. Moreover, despite the fact that surveys were mailed to the executive director of the agency, there is no way of knowing who within the organization actually completed the data collection instrument.

FUTURE DIRECTIONS, FURTHER STUDY

This study focused on the Open Systems model of the CVF as the most likely catalyzing force for driving an organization's engagement with advocacy activities. There are three remaining quadrants in the CVF for possible exploration and investigation in terms of their influence on advocacy activities in general and electronic advocacy activities specifically. It is possible that organizations operating from different quadrants of the model may value advocacy activities more highly or privilege advocacy activities as a mechanism for organizational stability differently from those found here. Future studies could compare how different quadrants of the CVF effect an organization's advocacy climate and level of engagement with advocacy activities.

Another logical next question is whether the embrace of the newer, digital age media results in more successful advocacy outcomes. Understanding the effectiveness of these new digital tools is imperative for preparing and educating future advocates entering the field, and is certainly important for individuals already practicing in the field. Human service organizations are not resource-rich institutions and frequently have little money or expertise to invest in their advocacy agendas. Actionable knowledge about the success of digital tools for meeting advocacy goals will be a real service to the sector and a boon in helping organizational leaders to make the appropriate and most efficient choices for their organizations.

REFERENCES

Almog-Bar, M., & Schmid, H. (2013). Advocacy activities of nonprofit human service organizations: A critical review. *Nonprofit and Voluntary Sector Quarterly 43*(7). Online publication. doi:10.1177/0899764013502584

Berry, J. M. (2005), Nonprofits and civic engagement. *Public Administration Review, 65*, 568–578. doi:10.1111/j.1540-6210.2005.00484.x

Berry, J. M., & Arons, D. F. (2003). *A voice for nonprofits.* Washington, DC: Brookings Institution.

Blackwood, A. (2012). *The nonprofit sector in brief: Public charities, giving and volunteering, 2012.* Washington, DC: The Urban Institute.

Bryant, A. (2006). Wiki and the Agora: "It's organizing, Jim, but not as we know it." *Development in Practice, 16*(6), 559–569.

Cameron, K. S., & Quinn, R. E. (2011). *Diagnosing and changing organizational culture: Based on the competing values framework.* San Francisco, CA: Jossey Bass.

Cameron, K. S., Quinn, R. E., DeGraff, J., & Thakor, A. V. (2006). Competing values leadership: Creating value in organizations. London, UK: Edward Elgar.

De Vita, C., Montilla, M., Reid, B., & Fatiregun, O. (2004). *Organizational factors influencing advocacy for children.* Washington, DC: Urban Institute Press.

Dillman, D. A. (2000). *Mail and Internet surveys: The tailored design method.* New York, NY: John Wiley.

Donaldson, L. P. (2007). Advocacy by nonprofit human service agencies: Organizational factors as correlates to advocacy behavior. *Journal of community Practice, 15*(3), 139–158.

FitzGerald, E., & McNutt, J. G. (1997). *Electronic advocacy in policy practice: A framework for teaching technologically based practice.* Paper presented at the 1997 CSWE Annual Program Meeting, Chicago.

Garrahan, P., & Stewart, P. (1992). *The Nissan enigma: Flexibility at work in a local economy.* London, UK: Mansell.

Germany, J. B. (Ed.). (2006). *Person to person to person: Harnessing the political power of on-line social networks and user generated content.* Washington, DC: The Institute for Politics, Democracy and the Internet, George Washington University.

Gibelman, M., & Kraft, S. (1996). Advocacy as a core agency program: Planning considerations for voluntary human service agencies. *Administration in Social Work, 20*(4), 43–59.

Gifford, B. D., Zammuto, R. F., & Goodman, E. A. (2002). The relationship between hospital unit culture and nurses' quality of work life. *Journal of Healthcare Management/American College of Healthcare Executives, 47*(1), 13.

Greenhalgh, R. G., MacFarlane, F., & Peacock, R. (2009). *Organizational factors influencing technology adoption and assimilation in the NHS: A systematic literature review.* London, UK: National Institute for Health Research Service Delivery and Organisation Programme.

Guo, C., & Saxton, G. (2014). Tweeting social change: How social media are changing nonprofit advocacy. *Nonprofit and Voluntary Sector Quarterly, 43*(1), 57–79.

Hager, M. A., Wilson, S., Pollak, T. H., & Rooney, P. M. (2003). Response rates for mail surveys of nonprofit organizations: A review and empirical test. *Nonprofit and Voluntary Sector Quarterly, 32*(2), 252–267.

Hartnell, C. A., Ou, A. Y., & Kinicki, A. (2011). Organizational culture and organizational effectiveness: A meta-analytic investigation of the competing values framework's theoretical suppositions. *Journal of Applied Psychology, 96*(4), 677.

Kalliath, T. J., Bluedorn, A. C., & Gillespie, D. F. (1999). A confirmatory factor analysis of the competing values instrument. *Educational and Psychological Measurement, 59*(1), 143–158.

Kanter, B., & Fine, A. (2010). *The networked nonprofit: Connecting with social media to drive change.* San Francisco, CA: Jossey Bass.

Khazanchi, S., Lewis, M. W., & Boyer, K. K. (2007). Innovation-supportive culture: The impact of organizational values on process innovation. *Journal of Operations Management, 25*(4), 871–884.

King, N., & Anderson, N. (1995). *Innovation and change in organizations.* London, UK: Routledge.

Kiesler, S., & Sproull, L. (1982). Managerial response to changing environments: Perspectives on problem sensing from social cognition. *Administrative Science Quarterly, 27*, 548–570.

Kimberlin, S. E. (2010). Advocacy by nonprofits: Roles and practices of core advocacy organizations and direct service agencies. *Journal of Policy Practice, 9*(3-4), 164–182.

Lawrence, K. A., Lenk, P., & Quinn, R. E. (2009). Behavioral complexity in leadership: The psychometric properties of a new instrument to measure behavioral repertoire. *The Leadership Quarterly, 20*(2), 87–102.

Macindoe, H., & Whalen, R. (2013). Specialists, generalists, and policy advocacy by charitable nonprofit organizations. *Journal of Sociology & Social Welfare, 40*(2), 119–149.

McNutt, J. (2007). Adoption of new-wave electronic advocacy techniques by nonprofit child advocacy organizations. In M. Cortes & K. Rafter (Eds.), *Nonprofits and technology: Emerging research for usable knowledge.* Chicago, IL: Lyceum.

McNutt, J. G., & Boland, K. M. (1999). Electronic advocacy by nonprofit organizations in social welfare policy. *Nonprofit and Voluntary Sector Quarterly, 28*(4), 432–451.

McNutt, J. G., & Menon, G. M. (2008). The rise of cyberactivism: Implications for the future of advocacy in the human services. *Families in Society: The Journal of Contemporary Social Services, 89*(1), 33–38.

Mosley, J. E. (2011). Institutionalization, privatization, and political opportunity: What tactical choices reveal about the policy advocacy of human service nonprofits. *Nonprofit and Voluntary Sector Quarterly, 40*(3), 435–457.

Nah, S., & Saxton, G. D. (2013). Modeling the adoption and use of social media by nonprofit organizations. *New Media & Society, 15*(2), 294–313.

O'Reilly, T. (2005). Web 2.0: Compact definition. Message posted to http://radar. oreilly. com/archives/2005/10/web_20_compact_definition.html

Ostroff, C., Kinicki, A. J., & Tamkins, M. M. (2003). Organizational culture and climate. *Handbook of psychology.* Wiley Online Library. doi:10.1002/0471264385.wei1222

Patterson, M. G., West, M. A., Shackleton, V. J., Dawson, J. F., Lawthom, R., Maitlis, S., . . . Wallace, A. M. (2005). Validating the organizational climate measure: Links to managerial practices, productivity and innovation. *Journal of Organizational Behavior, 26*(4), 379–408.

Quinn, R. E. (1988). *Beyond rational management*. San Francisco, CA: Jossey-Bass.

Quinn, R. E., & McGrath, M. R. (1985). The transformation of organizational cultures: A competing values perspective. In P. J. Frost & L. F. Moore (Eds.), *Organizational culture* (pp. 315–334). Beverly Hills, CA: Sage.

Quinn, R. E., & Rohrbaugh, J. (1981). A competing values approach to organizational effectiveness. *Public Productivity Review, 5*, 122–140.

Quinn, R. E., & Rohrbaugh, J. (1983). A spatial model of effectiveness criteria: Towards a competing values approach to organizational analysis. *Management Science, 29*(3), 363–377.

Roeger, K., Blackwood, A., & Pettijohn, S. (2012). *Nonprofit almanac 2012*. Washington, DC: Urban Institute Press.

Saidel, J. R., & Harlan, S. L. (1998). Contracting and patterns of nonprofit governance. *Nonprofit Management and Leadership, 8*(3), 243–259.

Salamon, L. M. (1995). Partners in public service: Government-nonprofit relations in the modern welfare state. Baltimore, MD: The Johns Hopkins University.

Schachter, H. L. (2011). Reflections on political engagement and voluntary association governance. *Nonprofit and Voluntary Sector Quarterly, 40*(4), 703–719.

Schein, E. H. (1983). The role of the founder in creating organizational culture. *Organizational Dynamics, 12*(1), 13–28.

Schein, E. H. (2006). *Organizational culture and leadership* (Vol. 356). San Francisco, CA: Jossey Bass.

Schneider, R. L., & Lester, L. (2001). *Social work advocacy: A new framework for action*. Belmont, CA: Brooks/Cole.

Smith, S. R., & Pekkanen, R. (2012). Revisiting advocacy by non-profit organizations. *Voluntary Sector Review, 3*(1), 35–49.

Suárez, D. F. (2009). Nonprofit advocacy and civic engagement on the Internet. *Administration & Society, 41*(3), 267–289.

Sumariwalla, R. D. (1986). *Toward a national taxonomy of exempt entities*. Washington, DC: Aspen Institute and United Way of America.

Tredinnick, L. (2006). Web 2.0 and Business: A pointer to the intranets of the future? *Business Information Review, 23*(4), 228–234.

West, M. A. (1996). Reflexivity and work group effectiveness: A conceptual integration. In M. A. West (Ed.), *Handbook of work group psychology* (pp. 555–579). Chichester, UK: Wiley.

West, M. A. (2000). Reflexivity, revolution, and innovation in work teams. In M. M. Beyerlein, D. A. Johnson, & S. T. Beyerlein (Eds.), *Product development teams* (pp. 1–29). Stamford, CT: JAI Press.

West, M. A., & Farr, J. L. (Eds.) (1990). *Innovation and creativity at work: Psychological and organizational strategies*. Chichester, UK: John Wiley & Sons.

Zafft, C., & Adams, S. (2008). *Applying the competing values framework to self-managed teams* (Master's thesis, American Society for Engineering Education). Retrieved from http://search.asee.org/search/fetch?url=file://localhost/E:/search/conference/12/2006Full2012.pdf&index=conference_papers&space=129746797203605791716676178&type=application/pdf&charset=

Zammuto, R. F., & O'Connor, E. J. (1992). Gaining advanced manufacturing technologies' benefits: The roles of organization design and culture. *Academy of Management Review, 17*(4), 701–728.

Identifying Attributes of Relationship Management in Nonprofit Policy Advocacy

NICOLE RUGGIANO
School of Social Work, Robert Stempel College of Public Health and Social Work, Florida International University, Miami, Florida, USA

JOCELYN DEVANCE TALIAFERRO
Department of Social Work, North Carolina State University, Raleigh, North Carolina, USA

FRANK R. DILLON
Division of Counseling and Psychology, School of Education, University at Albany – State University of New York, Albany, New York, USA

TED GRANGER
United Way of Florida, Tallahassee, Florida, USA

JESSICA SCHER
United Way of Miami-Dade, Miami, Florida, USA

Relationship management has been identified as an important activity for policy advocacy, but little is known about the strategies that human service administrators use to develop and maintain relationships with policymakers. This exploratory study aimed at identifying attributes of relationship management strategies that are associated with policy advocacy outcomes. Data were gathered from a sample of 333 nonprofit human service providers in Florida. Controlling for organizational size, the findings indicated that several established dimensions of relationship management were associated with policy advocacy success: networking, sharing of tasks, and assurances. Post hoc analyses found that the relationship between policy advocacy success and the domains of access and openness were respectively mediated by networking and sharing of tasks. Implications for nonprofit administrators and researchers are discussed.

Historically, policy advocacy has been a key function of the social work profession (Mosely, 2013), shaping American policy (Boris & Krehely, 2002) and linking community members with the public sphere (Frumkin, 2002). Social workers have an obligation to engage in policy advocacy (NASW, approved 1996, revised 2008), especially for those who are human service administrators, given that policy advocacy plays an important role in improving the social conditions of those seeking human services (Rome & Hoechstetter, 2010).

Evidence-based practice has been emphasized for social work overall, yet little is known about the best practices for policy advocacy. Indeed, Gen and Write (2013) have lamented that limited progress has been made at developing theory to guide policy advocacy practice. This is problematic given that social work administrators often need to balance the effort and resources required for advocacy with their organizations' larger demands. The literature suggests that relationship building plays an important role in nonprofit policy advocacy (Kovacs, 2001; Skinner, 2007), though there is a dearth of knowledge about the strategies that human service administrators utilize to cultivate relationships with policymakers and other nonprofit organizations for the purpose of attaining their policy advocacy goals. This exploratory study aimed at expanding current understandings about human service policy advocacy by identifying attributes of fostering and maintaining productive relationships within the context of policy advocacy activities.

POLICY ADVOCACY AS A HUMAN SERVICE ADMINISTRATIVE ACTIVITY

Policy advocacy is one of many political activities that nonprofit human service organizations engage in and may include direct or grassroots lobbying (Bass, Arons, Guinane, Carter, & Rees, 2007). Nonprofit human service administrators report that policy advocacy is an ongoing part of their management activities (Ruggiano & Taliaferro, 2012), though the extent to which organizations' are politically active varies (Bass et al., 2007). Research has identified a number of factors that influence an agency's likelihood to engage in political activities. It has been found that organizational capacity, access to technology, and staff dedicated to policy advocacy increase the likelihood that an organization will engage in policy advocacy (Bass et al., 2007; Suárez & Hwang, 2008), while restrictive government policies, knowledge of lobbying laws, lack of resources, lack of skills, and conservative policy environments curtail policy advocacy activities (Bass et al., 2007; Berry &

Arons, 2003; Frumkin, 2002; Mellinger & Kolomer, 2013; Salamon, Geller, & Lorentz, 2008).

Potential benefits abound for nonprofit human service organizations that participate in policy advocacy. From a macro perspective, policy advocacy allows organizations to facilitate systems-level change that benefits their constituents (Boris & Krehely, 2002; Frumkin, 2002). In addition, administrators have reported that their advocacy may result in a number of organizational benefits, including increasing public awareness; increasing funding for particular programs; protecting government programs that serve their constituents (Bass et al., 2007); and advancing their public service missions overall (Hessenius, 2007). Given these potential benefits, there is growing interest among human service administrators and researchers on the administrative and organizational behaviors that are related to policy advocacy.

The Role of Relationships in Policy Advocacy

Relationship management is one administrative activity that has received growing attention in the policy advocacy literature. Research has documented that building relationships with external stakeholders, such as policymakers and other nonprofit organizations, plays an important role in policy advocacy (deKieffer, 2007; Kovacs, 2001; Skinner, 2007). Human service organizations face significant competition with other self-interest groups when trying to attract the attention of policymakers (Teater, 2008). By building relationships with individual policymakers, human service administrators may make their issues more personal for policymakers, increase their credibility, and increase their access to policymakers (Kovacs, 2001; Teater, 2008) In addition, human service organizations may develop relationships with other organizations that have shared policy goals in an effort to strengthen their message and increase their capacity for policy advocacy (Ruggiano, Taliaferro, & Shtompel, 2013). Although the importance of relationship building has been acknowledged, research has not fully examined the relationship management strategies that nonprofit organizations utilize for the purpose of policy advocacy.

MANAGING RELATIONSHIPS

Relationship management has been used by scholars as a theoretical framework for studying organizations' efforts to develop and maintain relationships with their external stakeholders, often referred to as organizational-public relationships (OPRs). Ledingham and Brunning (1998, p. 62) define OPRs as "the state which exists between an organization and its key publics in which the actions of either entity impact the economic, social, political and/or cultural well-being of the other entity." Organizations that are effective at managing OPRs may have a positive effect on external stakeholders' attitudes, behaviors, and evaluation of the organization (Bruning, 2002; Bruning, Langenhop, & Green, 2004) and be more effective at attaining their goals (Dozier, Grunig, & Grunig, 1995). Research suggests that improving the quality of nonprofit OPRs may have numerous financial benefits to an organization, such as cultivating the pool of potential donors and increasing their likelihood of giving time and financial resources (Park & Rhee, 2010), retaining long-time donors (Sargeant, 2001), and obtaining new members (Banning & Schoen, 2007).

Human service organizations may be proactive at cultivating positive relationships with external stakeholders by utilizing relationship management strategies. Ki and Hon (2008, p. 5) define relationship management strategies as "any organizational behavioral efforts that attempt to establish, cultivate, and sustain relationships with strategic publics." Six strategies that are commonly the focus of organizational studies are access, positivity, openness, sharing of tasks, networking, and assurances (Bortree, 2010; Grunig & Huang, 2000; Ki & Hon, 2008; Park & Rhee, 2010). Ideally, by engaging in such behaviors, nonprofit human service organizations may strengthen their relationships with policymakers and other organizations that have similar policy agendas.

Access

Access refers to any strategy that an organization uses to engage an external stakeholder for sharing information, opinions, and thoughts (Ki & Hon, 2007). Ideally, organizations that want to develop stronger OPRs will provide their external stakeholders with increasing opportunities and outlets for bidirectional communication (Hon & Grunig, 1999). For the purpose of policy advocacy, we know that nonprofit organizations engage in a number of direct and grassroots activities aimed at engaging policymakers, including personally visiting with government officials, writing letters, telephoning, and using media outlets such as television and newspapers (Donaldson & Sheilds, 2009).

Openness

Access involves activities that provide opportunities for stakeholders to share information, thoughts, and feelings with the organization, whereas openness relates to the actual disclosure of information (Ki & Hon, 2007). This may involve the organization sharing information with stakeholders or encouraging its stakeholders to share information (Canary & Stafford, 1992). The information that is shared through openness goes beyond common knowledge. Ideally, this information should not be privy to others outside of the relationship or should relate to honest feelings and opinions regarding the parties involved (Ki & Hon, 2007). In terms of policy advocacy, openness may involve nonprofit human service organizations and policymakers discussing their thoughts and opinions about the need for policy or how specific policies are affecting service delivery or target populations (Donaldson & Sheilds, 2009).

Assurances

Assurance relates to "attempts by parties in the relationship to assure the other parties that they and their concerns are legitimate" (Hon & Grunig, 1999, p. 15). This may involve professing commitment and loyalty to external stakeholders (Canary & Stafford, 1992) or making sure that stakeholders know that the organization is addressing their concerns (Ki & Hon, 2007). Although policymakers acknowledge the value of interest groups in the decision-making process, they have a larger constituency that they are accountable to and therefore must balance interest groups' needs with the needs of their district (Teater, 2008). Therefore, nonprofit organizations may find greater chances of success by acknowledging and legitimizing policymakers' concerns so that a shared policy agenda may be developed, rather than an agenda that only meets the needs of the organization.

Networking

Networking relates to the level of effort that an organization exerts to develop alliances with other organizations that share similar stakeholders with which the organization would like to cultivate relationships (Ki & Hon, 2007). In the literature, networking for policy advocacy often involves collaborations among multiple organizations that have similar policy advocacy goals to strengthen their message and capacity to advocate (Donaldson & Sheilds, 2009).

Sharing of Tasks

Sharing of tasks is a relationship management strategy whereby an organization makes an effort to share responsibility in tasks or problem solving (Ki & Hon, 2007). These tasks and/or problems can be of mutual interest or separate between the organization and the stakeholder. Nonprofit organizations may actively involve a number of external stakeholders for the purpose of policy advocacy. One example can be seen through grassroots advocacy, where nonprofit organizations engage their constituents in contacting policymakers on issues affecting their services or community (Donaldson &

Sheilds, 2009). It may also involve joint advocacy efforts with other organizations within the nonprofit's network (Sherraden, Slosar, & Sherraden, 2002) or collaborative activities with policymakers (Mosley, 2011) in an attempt to work together to achieve policy-related goals to which all parties agree.

Positivity

The final relationship management strategy described by Hon and Grunig (1999) is positivity, which relates to organizational activities aimed at making the relationships with their stakeholders more enjoyable. For human service organizations, positivity may relate to the manner in which organizations respond to external stakeholders or their approach to address disagreements or problems experienced by one or more stakeholders (Park & Rhee, 2010).

EXPANDING OUR UNDERSTANDING OF RELATIONSHIP MANAGEMENT FOR POLICY ADVOCACY

Research indicates that relationships play a significant role in policy advocacy (Kovacs, 2001; Skinner, 2007) and that effective lobbying often requires organizations to develop and maintain relationships with decision makers (Kovacs, 2001; Richan, 2006). Prior studies on relationship management suggest that human service organizations that develop stronger and more positive relationships with policymakers and other external stakeholders for the purpose of policy advocacy may be more effective at achieving their policy advocacy goals. However, the use of relationship management strategies for the purpose of policy advocacy activity has remained primarily unexplored and there are currently no tools to measure the effectiveness of relationship management strategies for the purpose of policy advocacy.

The aim of this study is twofold. First, it sets out to identify specific theorized attributes of relationship management in policy advocacy among nonprofit human service organizations. Second, it intends to examine how these attributes relate to policy advocacy outcomes. To address these aims, we developed the following exploratory research questions:

1. What are attributes of relationship management strategies (access, openness, networking, assurances, sharing of tasks, and positivity) that are related to nonprofit policy advocacy?
2. How are these attributes of relationship management strategies related to policy advocacy success?

METHODS

This study was conducted in partnership with the United Way of Florida and United Way of Miami-Dade and involved an online survey of administers at nonprofit human service organizations in Florida. The methods and survey for this study were approved by the internal review board at Florida International University and have been reported elsewhere (Ruggiano, Taliaferro, Dillon, Granger, & Scher, 2014).

Procedure

Data were collected from local nonprofit human service organizations associated with a large intermediary organization with many statewide affiliates. The online survey was designed by a team of academics and administrators from the United Way of Florida and the United Way of Miami-Dade, which allowed for the construction of survey items that reflected both strong organizational management theory and practical knowledge. This process initiated with the researchers presenting the administrators with definitions of the relationship management strategies (Hon & Grunig, 1999; Ki & Hon, 2008), followed by a brainstorming session where the team devised an initial bank of items that reflected how nonprofit organizations utilize these strategies for the purpose of policy advocacy. The team also worked together to define "policy advocacy success" and generate a number of items that reflected successful outcomes for nonprofit organizations who engage in policy advocacy. After the initial item bank was generated, the team engaged in a process of reviewing, editing, and eliminating items based on their relevance and clarity. The team then piloted the final item bank by having three administrators from other nonprofit organizations complete the survey and provide feedback on their understanding and perceptions of the survey items. The team incorporated this feedback into a subsequent round of reviewing, editing, and item elimination.

The final survey items asked respondents about their organization's demographics and experience in relationship management, which included interacting with policymakers for the purpose of education or advocacy surrounding policy issues; and collaborating with other organizations and coalitions for the purpose of education or advocacy surrounding policy issues. The survey also asked questions about their organization's experience with achieving successful outcomes in policy advocacy/education.

The survey was distributed four times between April 2012 and August 2012 and used Qualtrics (Qualtrics Lab, Inc., 2013) online survey software to administer the survey and manage survey responses. To administer the survey the United Way of Florida sent an e-mail to administrators at its local affiliates across the state. The e-mail included an explanation of the survey, a link to the survey, a statement indicating that completing the survey implied consent to participate in the survey, and instructions to forward the e-mail to an administrator at each nonprofit organization that received funding through their organizations. No incentives were offered to participants.

Measures

No current measures exist for relationship management that are specific to policy advocacy. For the purpose of this study, relationship management strategies were defined using Hon and Grunig's (1999) identified strategies. These included access, openness, sharing of tasks, networking, assurances, and positivity.

Access. Access was defined as *any organizational attempts to engage policymakers and other nonprofit organizations for the purpose of policy advocacy* (Hon & Grunig, 1999). To measure access of participating organizations, participants were asked to respond to the level of frequency their organization engages in 11 behaviors, using a 6-point Likert-type scale (0 = *Never,* 3 = *Once a month,* 6 = *Once a Week*). Such behaviors included *personally visits government officials, telephones government officials, and e-mails government officials.* The *Access* composite score was obtained by summing scores from the 11 items yielding a range of 0–66. The Cronbach's alpha coefficient for the set of access items was .84.

Openness. Openness is defined as *any attempt by an organization to either share its thoughts and feelings about policy issues with policymakers and other nonprofit organizations or to encourage these stakeholders to share their thoughts and feelings about policy issues with the organization* (Hon & Grunig, 1999). *Openness* was measured by asking participants to respond to their level of agreement to 3 attitudes about organizational behavior, e.g., using a 5-point Likert-type scale (1 = *Strongly Disagree,* 3 = *Neutral,* 5 = *Strongly Agree*) and their level of frequency their organization *contacts government officials to learn about their opinions and thoughts regarding issues affecting our organization and community* using a 6-point Likert-type scale (0 = *Never,* 3 = *Once a month,* 5 = *Once a Week*). Examples of attitudinal items included *We share enough information with government officials about how policy issues affect our members* and *We share enough information with government officials about the programs and services we provide.* The *Openness* composite score was obtained by summing scores from the four items yielding a range of 3–20. The Cronbach's alpha coefficient for the set of openness items was .78.

Sharing of tasks. Sharing of tasks is defined as *organizational efforts aimed at initiating or accepting the sharing of responsibility with external stakeholders for policy advocacy and policy-related problem solving* (Hon & Grunig, 1999). To assess sharing of tasks, participants were asked to respond to their level of agreement to two items assessing attitudes about organizational behavior, e.g., using a 5-point Likert-type scale (1 = *Strongly Disagree*, 3 = *Neutral*, 5 = *Strongly Agree*) and their level of frequency their organization *contacts government officials to collaborate on projects that address problems affecting their organization/community* using a 6-point Likert-type scale (0 = *Never*, 3 = *Once a month*, 5 = *Once a Week*). Examples of attitudinal items included *Our organization engages constituents in educating government officials on policy issues affecting our organization and/or community* and *When we communicate to the public about the needs of our organization and the community, we emphasize the role that government officials play in addressing those needs*. A *Sharing of Tasks* composite score was obtained by summing scores from the three items yielding a range of 2–15. The Cronbach's alpha coefficient for the set of sharing of tasks items was .61.

Networking. Networking is defined as *organizational efforts aimed at developing alliances with other organizations that share similar policy advocacy goals* (Hon & Grunig, 1999). To assess networking, participants were asked to respond to three items. Two of the items, including *We contact other nonprofit organizations to discuss policy issues was measured* using a 5-point Likert-type scale (1 = *Strongly Disagree*, 3 = *Neutral*, 5 = *Strongly Agree*). The third item asked respondents to indicate the extent to which *working with other organizations to address our organization's policy goals* has been positive using a 5-point Likert-type scale (1 = *Extremely Negative*, 3 = *Neutral*, 5 = *Extremely Positive*). The *Networking* composite score was obtained by summing scores from the three items yielding a range of 3–15. The Cronbach's alpha coefficient for the set of networking items was .73.

Assurances. Assurance is defined as *organizational efforts aimed at acknowledging and legitimizing the concerns of policy makers* (Hon & Grunig, 1999). To assess assurances, participants were asked to respond to two items, using a 5-point Likert-type scale (1 = *Strongly Disagree*, 3 = *Neutral*, 5 = *Strongly Agree*). Sample items include *We make an effort to provide personal responses to government officials' concerns* and *We have a two-way relationship with government officials*. The *Assurances* composite score was obtained by summing scores from the two items yielding a range of 2–10. Internal consistency estimate was not calculated because of too few items (Tabachnick & Fidell, 2007).

Positivity. Positivity is defined as *organization' policy advocacy activities aimed at improving their existing relationships with external stakeholders* (Hon & Grunig, 1999). To assess positivity, participants were asked to respond to the question, *Networking with other organizations to engage in policy-related activities benefits our clients, members, and partners* using a 5-point Likert-type scale (1 = *Strongly Disagree*, 3 = *Neutral*, 5 = *Strongly Agree*).

Policy advocacy success. Policy advocacy success was used as an outcome measure and was measured by asking participants to respond to five items that indicated their organization's experience in participating in policy advocacy efforts that resulted in specific outcomes using a 5-point Likert-type scale (1 = *Strongly Disagree,* 3 = *Neutral,* 5 = *Strongly Agree*). The items developed to measure policy advocacy success were based on United Way administrators' perceptions of common goals that nonprofit human service organizations have for their policy advocacy activities. These identified goals were consistent with prior research on nonprofit advocacy (Nicholson-Crotty, 2009; Ruggiano & Taliferro, 2012). Sample items asked participants to indicate the extent to which they agreed that their organization participated in policy-related activities that have resulted in *increased funding for our organization, community, or partnering agencies* and *policies that positively affected how our organization provides services.* The *Policy Advocacy Success* composite score was obtained by summing scores from the five items yielding a range of 5–25. The Cronbach's alpha coefficient for the set of policy advocacy outcome items was .90.

Organizational size. Respondents were asked demographic questions regarding their organization's annual budget (coded as 1 = *Less than $25,000;* 2 = *$25,000–$99,999;* 3 = *$100,000–$249,000;* 4 = *$250,000–499,999;* 5 = *$500,000–$999,999,* 6 = *$1 million–$4,999,999,* 7 = *$5 million or more*).

Data Analysis

The first step in the analyses involved assessing the relationship management variables (access, openness, sharing of tasks, networking, positivity, and assurances) and the policy advocacy success outcome variable, as well as a demographic variable (organizational size) to determine if all variables violated the assumption of normality, based on Kline's (2005) suggestion of maximum absolute values of 3.0 for skewness and 8.0 for kurtosis. Then, correlations between all study variables were examined to assess the bivariate relationships among predictors, and initial estimates between hypothesized predictors and policy advocacy success. This also allowed for an analysis of potential multicollinearity among the variables, using Tabachnick and Fidell's (2007) recommended maximum values of correlation coefficients of less than .70. This was done by computing a correlation matrix among all study variables (see Table 1).

Finally, a hierarchical regression analysis was performed to examine the hypothesized relationship management predictors (access, openness, sharing of tasks, networking, and assurances) of nonprofit policy advocacy outcomes while accounting for organizational budget size. Organizational budget size was entered as the first block to control for potential differences in attributes due to organizational resources, which has been found in the research to

TABLE 1 Correlations Among Demographic, Predictor, and Criterion Variables ($N = 333$)

Variable	M	SD	1	2	3	4	5	6	7
1. Policy Advocacy Success	18.88	3.65	—						
2. Agency Budget Size	5.55	1.40	.36**	—					
3. Network	16.68	2.28	.39**	0.08	—				
4. Access	17.78	6.51	.29**	.14**	.23**	—			
5. Openness	13.58	3.15	.43**	.18**	.33**	.52**	—		
6. Assurances	4.39	1.43	−.49**	−.35**	−.32**	−.40**	−.49**	—	
7. Sharing of Tasks	8.77	2.27	.52**	.31**	.38**	.63**	.65**	−.62**	—

Note: $*p < .05$, $**p < .01$.

be a predictor of political activity for nonprofit organizations (Bass et al., 2007). Next, the hypothesized relationship management predictors were entered sequentially into the equation (access, openness, sharing of tasks, networking, and assurances) in order of increasing strength of their bivariate correlation with the outcome variable, policy advocacy success. This resulted in a total of six blocks in each regression model. (See Table 2).

RESULTS

Sample Characteristics

The survey was distributed to an estimated 1,034 nonprofit human service providers. There were 412 surveys completed; however, 78 cases were deleted due to missing predictor and/or outcome data, or duplicate IP addresses, which suggested multiple survey responses from the same agency. This resulted in a sample size of 333 and a response rate of 32.2%. Respondents represented organizations that were diverse and located across the state of Florida. The size of the organizations tended to be large. The annual operating budgets of the 303 participating organizations that provided budget information ranged from less than $25,000 to $5 million or more. Most respondents (35.3%) reported that their agency's budget was between $1 million and $4 million. The organizations reported a variety of missions, with family crisis (14.9%), school-age children (13.3%), and health (12.9%) being the most common missions.

Descriptive Statistics and Correlations

The bivariate correlation matrix revealed high multicollinearity between the independent variables *networking* and *positivity*, which were positively correlated with a Pearson correlation of 0.85. The research team determined that since the single item for *positivity* asked participants about their organization's participation in networks, it should be combined with the set of predictors for networking. The new set of four *networking* predictors had a

TABLE 2 Predictors of Policy Advocacy: Results of a Hierarchical Regression Model ($N = 333$)

Variable	B	SE B	β	t	R^2	ΔR^2	ΔF	Df
Step 1								
Agency Budget Size	0.79	0.13	0.30	5.85**	0.10	0.10	35.73**	1,338
Step 2								
Agency Budget Size	0.71	0.13	0.28	5.29**				
Access	0.14	0.03	0.26	5.19**	0.16	0.07	26.96**	2,337
Step 3								
Agency Budget Size	0.72	0.12	0.28	5.96**				
Access	0.10	0.03	0.18	3.76**				
Network	0.50	0.07	0.33	6.80**	0.26	0.10	46.10**	3,336
Step 4								
Agency Budget Size	0.72	0.12	0.28	5.87**				
Access	0.05	0.03	0.10	1.84				
Network	0.44	0.08	0.29	3.36**				
Openness	0.21	0.06	0.18	5.90**	0.29	0.02	10.75**	4,335
Step 5								
Agency Budget Size	0.60	0.12	0.23	4.89**				
Access	0.03	0.03	0.06	1.07				
Networking	0.40	0.07	0.26	5.37**				
Openness	0.16	0.06	0.14	2.45*				
Assurances	−0.51	0.14	−0.20	−3.64**	0.31	0.03	13.25**	5,334
Step 6								
Agency Budget Size	0.54	0.12	0.21	4.42**				
Access	−0.00	0.03	−0.01	−0.14				
Networking	0.36	0.08	0.23	4.76**				
Openness	0.10	0.07	0.08	1.46				
Assurances	−0.39	0.15	−0.15	−2.71**				
Sharing of Tasks	0.32	0.11	0.19	2.80**	.33	0.02	7.85*	6,333

Note: $*p < .05$, $**p < .01$.

Chronbach alpha of .82, which means that the addition of the *positivity* item increased the internal consistency of the *networking* dimension. The means, standard deviations, and bivariate correlation matrix of the other variables are presented in Table 1.

Hierarchical Regression Analysis

The results indicated that the overall set of predictors was highly related to policy advocacy outcomes, accounting for 32.4% of variability, $F(6, 339) = 27.14$, $p < 0.001$. Several hypothesized predictors were found to be significant in the final step of the model (see Table 2), which indicates that these variables had significant effects even when controlling for the other variables. These effects included *networking* (β = 0.35, $p < 0.001$), *sharing of tasks* (β = 0.29, $p < 0.05$), and *assurances* (β = −.44, $p < 0.01$).

It is important to note that both *access* (β = 0.07, $p < 0.05$) and *openness* (β = .16, $p < 0.05$) were found to be significant predictors in the third and fifth steps of the model, respectively. However, these predictors were not significant in the final step of the model ($\beta = -0.003$, $p = 0.94$ and $\beta = 0.11$, $p = 0.12$, respectively).

Post Hoc Mediation Analyses

The dimensions of access and openness were significantly related to policy advocacy outcomes when initially entered into the model, but were not significant in the final step of the hierarchical regression model. The bivariate correlation analysis (see Table 1) and an examination of changes in significance of predictors at each step of the hierarchical regression model suggested that networking may mediate the relationship between access and policy advocacy outcomes. Sharing of tasks also may mediate the relationship between openness and policy advocacy outcomes. Using a mediation test procedure based on bootstrap methods, analyses were performed using Mplus (Muthén & Muthén, 2007) statistical software to test the potential mediators (Shrout & Bolger, 2002). Five hundred bootstrap samples from the original data in each of the models were run to generate point estimates of the magnitude of the indirect effects and the associated 95% confidence intervals. If the confidence intervals exclude zero, then the indirect effects are statistically significant at the .05 level (Shrout & Bolger, 2002). Results from the mediation analyses demonstrated that relationship between access and outcome was significantly mediated by networking ($\beta = 0.08$, 95% confidence interval: 0.04—0.12) and that the relationship between openness and outcome was significantly mediated by sharing of tasks ($\beta = 0.28$, 95% confidence interval: 0.21—0.35).

DISCUSSION

Prior research has asserted that developing and maintaining relationships with policymakers play a role in policy advocacy (deKieffer, 2007; Kovacs, 2001; Richan, 2006; Skinner, 2007). However, little is known about the attributes of relationship management that are related to policy advocacy, resulting in a lack of best practices and assessment tools that can be used by social workers and researchers. To address this gap in knowledge, this study set out to examine if and how attributes of relationship management of human service administrators are associated with policy advocacy success.

A hierarchical regression analysis confirmed that three relationship management strategies are associated with policy advocacy: networking (developing alliances with organizations that share similar stakeholders with which the organization would like to cultivate relationships); assurances (making sure external stakeholders know that the organization is addressing their concerns); and sharing of tasks (share responsibility in tasks or problem solving). These findings are not surprising, given that prior research has indicated that relationship management strategies may increase a nonprofit's financial resources (Park & Rhee, 2010; Sargeant, 2001) and attract new members (Banning & Schoen, 2007). In addition, agency budget size was found to be associated with policy advocacy success, which was expected, given previous findings that organizational resources influence nonprofit organizations' political participation (deKieffer, 2007; Kovacs, 2001; Skinner, 2007).

The relationship between access and policy advocacy outcomes was significantly mediated by networking and the relationship between openness and policy advocacy outcomes was significantly mediated by sharing of tasks. These findings are also not surprising. Previous research on nonprofit networking has found that when advocacy groups have more cooperative relationships with government officials (which suggests an ongoing effort to network), the more opportunities they are given to have personal contact with those officials to express their opinions (Hoefer, 2005). Furthermore, policymakers are more likely to initiate contact with nonprofit administrators with whom they trust to gain information about policy-related decisions (Teater, 2008). In terms of interorganizational networking for the purpose of policy advocacy, when individual organizations strongly align themselves with a larger network/coalition, the interorganizational entity provides individual members with increased opportunities for contacting government officials (Ruggiano et al., 2013).

Research also sheds light on the finding that the relationship between openness and policy advocacy outcomes is mediated by sharing of tasks. Openness signifies a sense of trust between stakeholders that facilitates cooperation over time, though trust between stakeholders is constantly vulnerable (Edelenbos & Klijn, 2007). Therefore, it is possible that by sharing tasks with external stakeholders (government officials, other organizations, constituents, etc.) for the purpose of policy advocacy, nonprofit organizations' communications with external stakeholders are viewed as more meaningful and trusted. This may ultimately lead to higher probability of policy success.

Implications for Practitioners

These findings have several implications for practitioners. If nonprofit human service organizations are strategic in developing relationships with key government officials and other organizations for the purpose of policy advocacy, the strong relationships that develop may result in the human service organizations needing to exert less effort communicating with stakeholders in order to achieve success. Also, dividing tasks among stakeholders for the purpose of policy advocacy may strengthen the relationship between stakeholders, resulting in more effective communication. Essentially, nonprofit organizations can develop strategic communication plans as part of their policy goals that may result in policy advocacy becoming a more cost-effective organizational activity that still has a positive effect on their agency, services, and clients.

To accomplish these tasks, social workers should be strategic about their communication with policymakers that is ongoing, meaningful, and bi-directional (Bruning & Lambe, 2002). For instance, policy advocacy often involves practitioners and administrators communicating the needs of their organization and its clients to policymakers. However, policymakers are accountable to a larger constituency, and therefore they may view human service issues differently when placing them in the context of their larger constituency's demands. Social work administrators may improve their relationships with policymakers by making an effort to learn their policymakers' needs and their perspectives on human service provision, so that mutually beneficial goals may be developed. The findings also suggest that social work administrators should identify specific activities that their organization and policymakers can engage in to address these mutual goals. This sharing of tasks may help facilitate commitment, investment, and involvement in their organization's relationship with policymakers, which are key features of strong organizational-public relationships (Ledingham & Bruning, 1998). It is recommended that social work administrators engage in communication training specific to policy advocacy, so that they may develop the skills needed to relay information to policymakers in a way that is most receptive.

Implications for Research

This exploratory study identified specific attributes of relationship management that are associated with policy advocacy among nonprofit human services and examined how these attributes relate to policy advocacy outcomes. These findings may inform future research that could potentially lead to measures and best practices for policy practice. Such tools may be helpful for social work administrators so that they may target their policy advocacy efforts to those activities that are most likely to yield successful outcomes. Therefore, many of these findings should be further explored in future research.

The limitations to this study should be considered when interpreting the results. First, it is important to note that this was not a random sample of nonprofit human service agencies. The organizations that participated in this survey were not representative of the larger population of nonprofit human service providers in that they tended to have large budgets and only provide services in Florida. The potential for social desirability bias in participants' reporting should also be noted. Since respondents represented United Way affiliates and organizations that partner with the United Way, it is possible that they may have felt pressure to over-report their policy advocacy activities and/or level of achieved success. However, the survey was designed to minimize such bias by allowing anonymous and voluntary responses. In addition, the expected positive correlation between the construct *policy advocacy success* and organizational budget size suggests that social desirability bias did not have a significant impact on the responses.

There were also limitations stemming from how the theoretical constructs were measured. Without established definitions and measures for "policy advocacy relationship management," this study modified and evaluated existing definitions of access, openness, networking, sharing of tasks, positivity, and assurances to create items for the survey. Future studies should consider further examining how these dimensions should be defined and measured within the context of policy advocacy. There is a particular need to further explore how assurances and sharing of tasks should be measured, since these dimensions were determined to have low internal consistency in the current study. Future studies should attempt to identify a larger number of items to better assess these dimensions.

Similarly, future work should examine the theoretical dimension of positivity. Given the high degree of overlap between the item assessing positivity and the networking scale, the research team decided to combine the two dimensions, resulting in a four-item networking dimension. Although positivity was not distinctly included in the analysis, Hon and Grunig (1999, p. 13) assert that "not all strategies for maintaining relationships are equally effective. ... Therefore, we must recognize that not all public relations strategies, techniques, and programs are equally likely to produce relationship outcomes." Given administrators' difficulty in conceptualizing positivity during the item generation process, it is possible that this is not an effective strategy for the purpose of policy advocacy. Despite these limitations, this research successfully identified relationship management as a theoretical framework and administrative activity associated with policy advocacy outcomes.

Research should also further explore other ways that relationship management plays a role in human service organizations' advocacy behaviors. For instance, given the benefits of including constituents in advocacy activities (Lombe & Sherraden, 2008), research should further examine how relationship management is used to engage clients and supporters in policy advocacy. In addition, Mellinger's (2014) work highlights the importance of non-legislative advocacy among organizations. Therefore, research should explore how relationship management may relate to other types of advocacy efforts among human service organizations.

Conclusions

Policy advocacy has remained an important activity within the field of social work. This study contributes to the existing body of knowledge on policy practice by highlighting the importance of developing and maintaining meaningful relationships between nonprofit human service administrators and policymakers. It also furthers the discussion of developing theory for guiding policy practice (Gen & Write, 2013). By building upon these findings, it may be possible to make policy advocacy a more accessible and efficient activity within the nonprofit sector.

REFERENCES

Banning, S. A., & Schoen, M. (2007). Maximizing public relations with the organization–public relationship scale: Measuring a public's perception of an art museum. *Public Relations Review, 33,* 437–439.

Bass, G. D., Arons, D. F., Guinane, K., Carter, M. F., & Rees, S. (2007). *Seen but not heard. Strengthening nonprofit advocacy.* Washington, DC: The Aspen Institute.

Berry, J. M., & Arons, D. F. (2003). *A voice for nonprofits.* Washington, DC: Brookings Institution Press.

Boris, E. T., & Krehely, J. (2002). Civic participation and advocacy. In L. M. Salamon (Ed.), *The state of nonprofit America* (pp. 299–330). Washington, DC: The Brookings Institution Press.

Bortree, D. S. (2010). Exploring adolescent–organization relationships: A study of effective relationship strategies with adolescent volunteers. *Journal of Public Relations Research, 22,* 1–25.

Bruning, S. D. (2002). Relationship building as a retention strategy: Linking relationship attitudes and satisfaction evaluations to behavioral outcomes. *Public Relations Review, 28,* 39–48.

Bruning, S. D., & Lambe, K. (2002). Relationship building and behavioral outcomes: Exploring the connection between relationship attitudes and key constituent behavior. *Communication Research Reports, 19,* 327–337.

Bruning, S. D., Langenhop, A., & Green, K. A. (2004). Examining city–resident relationships: Linking community relations, relationship building activities, and satisfaction evaluations. *Public Relations Review, 30,* 335–345.

Canary, D. J., & Stafford, L. (1992). Relational maintenance strategies and equity in marriage. *Communication Monographs, 59,* 239–267.

deKieffer, D. E. (2007). *The citizen's guide to lobbying Congress.* Chicago, IL: Chicago Review Press, Inc.

Donaldson, L. P., & Sheilds, J. (2009). Development of the policy advocacy behavior scale: Initial reliability and validity. *Research on Social Work Practice, 19,* 83–92.

Dozier, D. M., Grunig, L. A., & Grunig, J. E. (1995). *Manager's guide to excellence in public relations and communication management.* Mahwah, NJ: Lawrence Erlbaum Associates.

Edelenbos, J., & Klijn, E. (2007). Trust in complex decision-making networks: A theoretical and empirical exploration. *Administration & Society, 39,* 25–50.

Frumkin, P. (2002). *On being nonprofit. A conceptual and policy primer*. Cambridge, MA: Harvard University Press.

Gen, S., & Wright, A. C. (2013). Policy advocacy organizations: A framework linking theory and practice. *Journal of Policy Practice, 12*, 163–193.

Grunig, J. E., & Huang, Y.-H. (2000). From organizational effectiveness to relationship indicators: Antecedents of relationships, public relations strategies, and relationship outcomes. In J. A. Ledingham & S. D. Bruning (Eds.), *Public relations as relationship management: A relational approach to the study and practice of public relations* (pp. 23–53). Mahwah, NJ: Lawrence Erlbaum Associates.

Hessenius, B. (2007). *Hardball lobbying for nonprofits. Real advocacy for nonprofits in the new century*. New York, NY: Palgrave MacMillan.

Hoefer, R. (2005). Altering state policy: Interest group effectiveness among state-level advocacy groups. *Social Work, 50*, 219–227.

Hon, L. C., & Grunig, J. E. (1999). *Guideline for measuring relationships in public relations*. Gainesville, FL: Institute for Public Relations. Retrieved from http://www.instituteforpr.org/files/uploads/Guidelines_Measuring_Relationships.pdf

Ledingham, J. A., & Bruning, S. D. (1998). Relationship management in public relations: Dimensions of an organization-public relationship. *Public Relations Review, 24*, 55–65.

Lombe, M., & Sherraden, M. (2008). Inclusion in the policy process: An agenda for participation of the marginalized. *Journal of Policy Practice, 7*, 199–213.

Ki, E. J., & Hon, L. C. (2007, May). *Reliable and valid relationship maintenance strategies measurement*. Paper presented at the annual meeting of the International Communication Association, San Francisco, CA.

Kline, R. B. (2005). *Principles and practice of structural equation modeling* (2nd ed.). New York, NY: Guilford Press.

Kovacs, R. (2001). Relationship building as integral to British activism: Its impact on accountability in broadcasting. *Public Relations Review, 27*, 421–436.

Mellinger, M. S. (2014). Beyond legislative advocacy: Exploring agency, legal, and community advocacy. *Journal of Policy Practice, 13*, 45–58.

Mellinger, M. S., & Kolomer, S. (2013). Legislative advocacy and human service nonprofits: What are we doing? *Journal of Policy Practice, 12*, 87–106.

Mosley, J. E. (2011). Institutionalization, privatization, and political opportunity: What tactical choices reveal about the policy advocacy of human service nonprofits. *Nonprofit and Voluntary Sector Quarterly, 40*, 435–457.

Mosley, J. E. (2013). The beliefs of homeless service managers about policy advocacy: Definitions, legal understanding, and motivations to participate. *Administrative Social Work, 37*, 73–89.

Muthén, L., K., & Muthén, B. O. (1998–2007). *Mplus user's guide* (5th ed.). Los Angeles, CA: Muthén & Muthén.

National Association of Social Workers (NASW). (approved 1996, revised 2008). *Code of Ethics*. Retrieved from http://socialworkers.org/pubs/code/code.asp

Nicholson-Crotty, J. (2009). The stages and strategies of advocacy among nonprofit reproductive health providers. *Nonprofit and Voluntary Sector Quarterly, 38*, 1044–1053.

Park, H., & Rhee, Y. (2010). Associations among relationship maintenance strategies, organisation-public relationships, and support for organisations: An exploratory study of the non-profit sector. *PRism 7*(2). Retrieved from http://praxis.massey.ac.nz/fileadmin/Praxis/Files/Journal_Files/Park_Rhee.pdf

Qualtrics Labs, Inc. (2013). *Qualtrics*. Provo, UT: Author.

Richan, W. C. (2006). *Lobbying for social change* (3rd ed.). Binghamton, NY: Haworth Press, Inc.

Rome, S. H., & Hoechstetter, S. (2010). Social work and civic engagement: The political participation of professional social workers. *Journal of Sociology & Social Welfare, 37*, 107–129.

Ruggiano, N., & Taliaferro, J. D. (2012). Resource dependency and agent theories: A framework for exploring nonprofit leaders' resistance to lobbying. *Journal of Policy Practice, 11*(4), 219–235.

Ruggiano, N., Taliaferro, J. D., Dillon, F., Granger, T., & Scher, J. (2014). Networking for policy advocacy: Identifying predictors of advocacy success among human service organizations. *Human Services Organizations Management, Leadership & Governance, 38*, 89–102.

Ruggiano, N., Taliaferro, J. D., & Shtompel, N. (2013). Interorganizational partnerships as a strategy for lobbying: Nonprofit administrators' perspectives on collaborating for systems-level change. *Journal of Community Practice, 21*, 263–281.

Salamon, L. M., Geller, S. L., & Lorentz, S. C. (2008). *Nonprofit America. A force for democracy?* (Communiqué #9). Baltimore, MD: Johns Hopkins University Center for Civil Society Studies.

Sargeant, A. (2001). Relationship fundraising: How to keep donors loyal. *Nonprofit Management & Leadership, 12*, 177–192.

Sherraden, M. S., Slosar, B., & Sherraden, M. (2002). Innovation in social policy: Collaborative policy advocacy. *Social Work, 47*, 209–221.

Shrout, P. E., & Bolger, N. (2002). Mediation in experimental and nonexperimental studies: New procedures and recommendations. *Psychological Methods, 7*, 422–445.

Skinner, R. M. (2007). *More than money. Interest group action in congressional elections*. Lanham, MD: Rowman & Littlefield.

Suárez, D. F., & Hwang, H. (2008). Civic engagement and nonprofit lobbying in California, 1998–2003, *Nonprofit and Voluntary Sector Quarterly, 37*, 93–112.

Tabachnick, B. G., & Fidell, L. S. (2007). *Using multivariate statistics* (5th ed.). Boston, MA: Allyn and Bacon.

Teater, B. (2008). "Your agenda is our agenda": State legislators' perspectives of interest group influence on political decision making. *Journal of Community Practice, 16*, 201–220.

Advocacy Tactics and Policy Outcomes of Sex Offender Rights Organizations

ERIN COMARTIN
Department of Sociology, Anthropology, Social Work & Criminal Justice, Oakland University, Rochester, Michigan, USA

Social movement organizations for sex offender rights work to reduce harm to registrants and their family members by influencing sex offender registration and community notification policies. This study draws on two theories of social movement organizations—organizational emergence and political opportunities—to investigate the capacity (i.e., structure, resources, knowledge and skills) of these organizations to bring about policy changes. Data were gathered using in-depth, telephone interviews with 19 leaders of state-level advocacy organizations in the United States. Two types of strategies emerged, distinguishing organizations as proactive or reactive in their approach to policy change. Proactive organizations contribute to policy amendment, development or adoption, whereas reactive organizations focus on blocking policy. These two types of organizations have similar tactical repertoires; however, more proactive organizations report the use of networking and coalition building and media stories, and more reactive organizations report the use of legislative testimony and research and policy analysis tactics. This study informs social work policy and practice by highlighting effective and ineffective tactics used by highly stigmatized advocacy organizations.

BACKGROUND

Social movement organizations (SMOs) have emerged across the country to change sex offender registration and notification (SORN) legislation, called anti-SORN SMOs in this study. These policies mandate that individuals charged with a sex crime have to periodically register with the police in order to provide their personal information and photograph. Police departments then put this information on an Internet-based registry for the public to view. By having this information viewable to the public, registrants have been subjected to harassment and isolation and have also lost employment and housing (Tewksbury, 2005). The resulting consequences also extend to registrants' family members (Levenson & Tewksbury, 2009). It is these unintended consequences that most often motivate offenders and their family members to organize for change.

In this study, I examine the rise of these organizations and their attempts to make state-level policy change. Drawing on interviews with 19 leaders of anti-SORN SMOs, my goal is to understand the resources and tactics of these organizations to bring about change in the political arena. To do so, I ask the following questions: What organizational factors, including structure, resources, knowledge, and skill, are associated with anti-SORN SMOs reporting successful achievement of a policy outcome? How do these organizational factors, along with the political environment, shape the strategy and tactics used to achieve a policy outcome? This study is guided by social movement concepts relating to organizational emergence along with political process/political opportunity theories.

The results show that anti-SORN SMOs have a moderate level of formalization, few material resources, and varying levels of human capital. What appears to be the most challenging resource for these organizations is obtaining organizational legitimacy perceived by policymakers and the media. It is this relationship with the political and media environments that shapes organizational strategy into either proactive or reactive stances. While these organizations have a range of SORN policy knowledge and have the basic advocacy skill set, some key areas of knowledge and skill are missing. In addition, anti-SORN SMOs are unlikely to use tactics used in other movements, such as rallies and marches, because the stigma attached to sex offenders draws public attention to the issue. I find that anti-SORN SMOs rarely change their tactics to adapt to the quick-changing focus of the political environment; however, they use political opportunities to their advantage when available.

As a profession, social workers generally hold more sympathy for victims of sex crimes than perpetrators, when compared to other professionals involved in cases of sexual violence (Saunders, 1988). However, the profession's values for the entitlement of basic human rights (Council on Social

Work Education, 2008) and dignity and worth of the person (National Association of Social Workers, 2008) suggest that social workers address social injustices, even for individuals who are morally responsible for their marginalization in society (Geiger, 2006). Thus, this article fills many gaps within the social work literature. At the micro level, individuals and families are experiencing physical, psychological, and social harms in their daily functioning from registration and community notification policies. At the macro level, this study represents a grassroots movement of marginalized voices, whereby the coordination of resources through organizational structures is working to change public policy. Thus, social work practitioners may come to understand effective and ineffective tactics used in advocacy work with offender based, and other types of stigmatized populations.

SORN Policies

In 1990, the State of Washington instituted the first SORN policy (Terry & Ackerman, 2009). From this policy, federal and state policies spread across the country, resulting in various forms of SORN policies in each jurisdiction. The federal policies that guide the adoption of state policies are based on the Jacob Wetterling Act of 1994, Megan's Law of 1996 and the Adam Walsh Act of 2006 (Logan, 2009). Ultimately, these policies led to the creation of publicly available, Internet-based registries, in which an offender's picture, home address, criminal charge, and personal identifying information is placed for public viewing. As of 2011, there were 747,408 registered sex offenders in the United States (The National Center for Missing and Exploited Children, 2011). Multiplying this number by the average family household size in 2010 of 2.58 (U.S. Census Bureau, 2012), it is likely that the policy affects approximately 1.9 million individuals.

Research regarding the consequences of SORN laws has found that registrants endure harassment, violence, and in some rare cases, homicide, because of public registration (Human Rights Watch, 2007; Levenson, D'Amora, & Hern, 2007). Registered sex offenders also report feelings of isolation, stigmatization, and an overall feeling of vulnerability (Tewksbury & Lees, 2006). These feelings increase their level of stress, which is believed to lead to re-offense (Levenson, 2008). In addition to these psychosocial harms, in a study of 121 registrants, many reported the loss of employment (43%) and housing (45%) as a result of having their name and address on the public registry (Tewksbury, 2005). Housing difficulties of registrants have resulted from policies that mandate their residence to be outside a specified distance from schools, daycare centers, and parks (Levenson, 2008). This causes registrants to live in less desirable neighborhoods (Grubesic, Mack, & Murray, 2007) or to become homeless (Levenson, 2008), which presents barriers for access to treatment and parole or probation meetings. Studies have shown that these collateral consequences for those who are mandated to register are likely to impede an offender's reintegration into society when compared to offenders that do not have to register (Tewksbury, Jennings, & Zgoba, 2012).

Collateral consequences extend to the individuals who live with a registrant. Individuals who are related to, or share the same address posted on the public registry, have lost housing they owned or rented because the property owner or a neighbor found out that a registrant was living at the address (Levenson & Tewksbury, 2009). Family members have also experienced social and psychological consequences from having a member listed on the registry such as feelings of shame, isolation from friends and family, and helplessness or hopelessness about the situation (Comartin, Kernsmith, & Miles, 2010).

SORN policies have been legally challenged in both federal and state court systems in regards to their agreement with the U.S. and State Constitutions. Challenges to these policies have been made on the constitutional grounds of freedom from cruel and unusual punishment, prohibition of ex post facto, equal protection of the law, right to privacy, right to travel, and due process of the law (Finn, 1997; Lewis, 1996; Mancini & Mears, 2013). In most cases, defendants argue multiple constitutional rights violations, with some arguments rejected by the court while others are successfully challenged (Mancini & Mears, 2013). Most arguments are rejected by the court (Logan, 2009), generally noting that the requirements are not a form of punishment (*Smith v. Doe*, 2003). However, in 2010 the Ohio State Supreme Court (*State v. Williams*) found registration and notification policies to be punitive in nature. When courts find policies to be unconstitutional, the goal is to have legislators amend the policy to make it constitutional (Van Horn, Baumer, & Gromley, 2001). In the Ohio case, this resulted in high costs to the state to implement a new policy, only for it to subsequently be found unconstitutional, which called for additional money spent to return to the original policy. The challenged constitutionality of SORN policies, along with the exorbitant costs to states, creates an opportunity for the anti-SORN movement to mobilize for policy change.

Anti-SORN Movement and SMOs

In reaction to the collateral consequences and constitutional rights violations felt by registrants, groups comprised of registrants, their family members, and professionals from the criminal justice and treatment fields have mobilized to create organizations that are focused on amending or eliminating SORN policies. Building on the work of Leon (2011), I argue that the emergence of these organizations is an indicator of a growing anti-SORN movement made up of state-level SMOs. These anti-SORN groups include individuals with shared values who work to support the group's cause (Hoefer, 2006) or who attempt to change a policy by using a variety of resources and tactics to achieve their desired policy outcomes (Davis, McAdam, Scott, & Zald, 2006). SMOs may propose new alternatives to current policies, or they may attempt to block policies that deter progress toward their goals (Kingdon, 2003).

Drawing on Whittier's (2009) analysis of the movement against child sexual abuse, I move this analysis from the realm of understanding this issue as a social problem in response to a "moral panic" (Jenkins, 1998) to conceptualizing anti-SORN efforts as a movement made up of sustained efforts challenging state policies through the endeavors of organizations, networks, and individuals (see Leon, 2011 and Whittier, 2009). The anti-SORN movement has grown from a few individuals talking to their legislators to incorporated organizations that operate to help registrants and their families navigate the criminal justice system and mobilize these individuals to advocate for policy change. Many in the movement have built networks with other justice-focused organizations, such as offender re-entry groups and victims' rights organizations (Leon, 2011). Anti-SORN organizations are mobilized to attempt policy changes, and their success depends on the political opportunity structure and its openness to change (McCarthy, 1996; Tarrow, 1996). As Whittier (2009, p. 15) noted, "Ties to policymakers, major institutions, sources of funding, and knowledge production affect activists' ability to form organizations and make social change." By bringing a social movement perspective to this issue, I focus on the activists, their view of the need for change, and the routes they take to affect it. I first focus on the theories of organizational emergence and then how these organizations operate in, and are shaped by, their environment. I conclude by discussing the way in which policy change is affected.

Organizational theory. Theories of organizational emergence focus on the process and structures within the organization (McAdam & Scott, 2005) and specifically investigate how organizational arrangements have either increased or decreased the organization's ability to survive and bring about social change (Buechler, 1995). Zald and Ash (1966) found that, over time, organizations became legitimate entities as they accumulated resources and built hierarchical structures to conduct the work needed to sustain a social movement and to further mobilize their members. Furthermore, Edwards and McCarthy (2007) found that not only is mobilization of the members important, but the knowledge and skills that they bring to the organization's endeavors are critical to meeting the organization's goals. The availability of resources for collective action is a dominant focus of SMOs, as they are generally operating with insufficient resources, especially organizations in the earlier phases of development (Zald & Ash, 1966). Organizational emergence also focuses on organizational structure. In many cases SMOs can expect change as they accumulate greater resources (e.g., time, skill, money) as opposed to a decentralized structure with inclusive membership and few professional staff members (McAdam & Scott, 2005).

Meshing with theories of political opportunities, Zald and Ash (1966) argued that movement organizations are influenced by the environment in which they operate, which suggests a dynamic relationship whereby organizations achieve greater outcomes when they adapt to the constraints placed on them by the environment (McAdam & Scott, 2005).

Therefore, anti-SORN SMOs' relationship to the political environment is crucial to their success. One barrier exists for this movement that is not as prevalent in other social movements: the stigma associated with the sex offender population. To counteract this barrier, it is imperative for anti-SORN SMOs to have a skilled and knowledgeable membership and a semi-structured hierarchy that is efficient and effective at negotiating with policymakers and the public regarding these issues.

Political opportunity theory. SMOs can be constrained by competing organizations or the government when their associated interests begin to conflict (McPhail, 1991). Tilly and Rule (1965) emphasized the importance of an organization's opportunities to pursue its interests and the impact that powerful decision makers have on the organization's level of effectiveness. Political opportunities can mobilize a social movement and affect the tactics that organizations employ to accomplish their policy strategies in a variety of ways. First, the relative openness of a political system, which determines if voices of the public are included in political decision making, will determine if an organization is able to play a role in the policy process. Second, the stability or instability of the political alignments that are operating at any given time within the political system, such as partisanship, are also likely to determine how an organization chooses to align itself to gain access to key decision makers. Third, organizations are more likely to be heard if they have elites as supporters of their cause, such as long-term politicians or the heads of bureaucratic institutions (McAdam, 1994; Tarrow, 1996). Anti-SORN SMOs exist in political environments that have only recently become open to the voices of sex offenders and their family members, based on the constitutional challenges and costs to maintain the registry. In addition, they are competing for the attention of policymakers with individuals and organizations that have different interests, such as victims' rights organizations or the justice system, at a time of polarized politics. The existence of policy elites who are willing to advocate for this issue may or may not exist. These constraints and opportunities are likely to affect the work undertaken by anti-SORN SMOs.

Policy change is a difficult and long-term process (Rothenberg, 1992), thus the focus of many SMOs is on shorter-term outcomes including an increase in the organization's capacity to change policy and minor changes in the political arena. Shorter-term policy change can include bringing awareness to the issue with policymakers or the public (Reisman, Gienapp, & Stachowiak, 2007). Members of the organizations focus on two types of tactics for change: those related to the political arena and those related to outreach. The Harvard Family Research Project (HFRP) (2009) describes the various tactics that advocacy organizations use to change policy. Tactics in the political arena include analysis and research, education, legal advocacy, proposal development, lobbying, and building relationships with decision makers (HFRP, 2009). For outreach, members may be involved in coalition and network building, grassroots mobilization, rallies and marches, voter education, public service announcements and other forms of media engagement, electronic social media campaigns, briefings, testimony, presentations on the issue, demonstration projects or pilot programs, and polling advocacy (HFRP, 2009). Anti-SORN SMOs are likely to use both short- and long-term tactics that focus on the political arena and outreach, all of which are dependent on the capacity of the organization. In addition, Kingdon (2003) suggests that opportunities for significant policy changes are likely to occur suddenly and that the window of opportunity will be open only a short time. To achieve the ultimate policy goal, SMOs must be ready with a well-developed policy proposal that is technically, financially, and politically acceptable to decision makers. Thus, anti-SORN SMOs must have a fully articulated plan ready when a window of opportunity presents itself.

METHODS

Nineteen interviews were conducted for this study. I used the website *Reform Sex Offender Laws (RSOL)* as the sampling frame because it was the only publicly available listing of anti-SORN SMOs. RSOL is a national organization that links the state organizations together. The website had a page that listed the e-mail addresses for 39 leaders of RSOL state affiliate organizations. In addition, a snowball sampling method (Rubin & Babbie, 2010) was used to gain further participants by asking interviewees to provide information for leaders of other anti-SORN SMOs that were conducting similar policy change efforts in other states. Snowball sampling was particularly useful as a recruitment strategy because of the stigma associated with this topic. For states where no organizations could be found through RSOL, an attempt to recruit leaders was made by contacting the state affiliates of two different organizations, The Association for the Treatment of Sexual Abusers and the Department of Corrections, to determine if they were aware of anti-SORN SMOs in their respective states.

The anti-SORN SMOs were operating in states from each region of the country (U.S. Census Bureau, 2011) and from states in all four quantiles of states ranked by total population (U.S. Census Bureau, 2010). Organizations were split evenly by political partisanship of the state, with nine representing Republican states and ten representing Democratic states (Newman, 2012). In addition, there was participation from anti-SORN SMOs in states with the highest (300 or more per 100,000 state population), middle (200 to 299 per 100,000 state population) and lowest (199 or fewer per 100,000 state population) per capita rates of registered sex offenders (National Center for Missing and Exploited Children, 2011). At the time that the interviews were conducted, fifteen states across the country had substantially complied with the Adam Walsh Act of 2006 (Office of Sex Offender Sentencing, Monitoring, Apprehending, Registering, and Tracking, 2011). Organizations from five of these 15 states participated in the study. Conversely, anti-SORN SMOs from two states that have publicly objected to compliance with this act also participated in the study (Clark, 2012; see updates at National Conference of State Legislatures, 2012). Thus, the anti-SORN SMO leaders who participated in this study are likely to represent various experiences with SORN policies.

I created the interview instrument, and the first version was piloted one year prior to this study with 12 leaders of RSOL organizations. Substantial changes were made to the instrument based on the findings from these preliminary interviews, and a second version of the instrument was piloted with one leader from another anti-SORN SMO. Once this leader verified that the questions were applicable and understandable based on the work of her organization, the final interview instrument was complete and was used with all 19 organizations that participated in this study.

After the institutional review board approved the final instrument (Protocol# 1109010163), an e-mail was sent to each leader listed on the RSOL website (39) to request their participation in this study. Interested individuals were asked to contact the researcher to participate. Seventeen leaders responded through this e-mail solicitation, with two additional interviews found through snowball sampling. Interviews were held between October 2011 and January 2012. Interviews lasted anywhere from one to four hours, depending on the depth of information provided by the interviewee. The trustworthiness of each interview was determined if the leader was able to articulate the resources, tactics, and outcomes of the organization and, over the course of the interviews, when responses to questions were saturated (Glaser & Strauss, 1967). All of the interviews were audio recorded and transcribed. The transcribed documents were sent to each corresponding participant for member checking (Creswell & Miller, 2000), which gave participants the opportunity to verify that the transcriptions accurately reflected their statements and intentions. Feedback that these participants provided was incorporated into the transcript because the comments were considered to add more trustworthiness to the responses.

The interview instrument included questions under three major themes: organizational factors, policy outcomes, and the tactics perceived to influence a successful policy outcome. Organizational factors included questions about the formalization of the organization (i.e., incorporation, hierarchy, task delegation, and written documents), material resources by proxy of an operating budget, the knowledge regarding SORN policies and the advocacy skills of the membership. (See Appendix A for the lists of knowledge and skills queried in the interview guide.) Regarding the policy outcome achieved, interviewees were asked, "Can you tell me about the best example of a successful policy outcome in your organization's history?" Interviewees were provided with a list of potential policy outcomes (see Appendix B for list of outcomes, drawn from HFRP, 2009.) Organizations could have succeeded in many policy outcomes throughout the organization's history, but this analysis focuses on the one that they believed to have the most impact on their ultimate goals. Once the interviewees described their most successful policy outcome, they were asked to talk about the tactics they used that were likely to influence the achievement of this outcome (list was drawn from HFRP, 2009). To garner information about opportunities in the political environment interviewees were asked, "Thinking about the policy outcome your organization was able to achieve, was something happening in the political arena or the media at the time that influenced the outcome?" They were then probed about politics by asking about events occurring around elections, change of leadership in government positions, or relationships between politicians. Another probe asked about the use of any sympathetic cases in the media. Finally, they were asked if they used any court case rulings to persuade policymakers on this issue. Interviewees could have used more than one opportunity in conjunction with their achieved policy outcome. Interviewees were asked about adapting to the environment through one question, "Has a situation arisen where you were going to employ an advocacy tactic but the organization changed the tactic?" Leaders were probed with follow-up questions about the reason for the change and the result of the change in tactic.

The data were coded in NVivo 9 through the use of "open coding", which describes the overall themes found within the data (Strauss & Corbin, 1990). Once open coding was finalized, some data were transformed into three numeric indices: formalized structure, SORN policy knowledge, and advocacy skills. Formalized structure is an index that ranges from zero to 18, with a higher score meaning a more formalized structure. This index was created by assigning a 1 if the organization reported the following elements and a zero if they did not: incorporation of the organization, having an identified leader, having an executive team, holding business meetings, leadership/executive team decisionmaking. The index was creating by summing these elements, along with the number of written documents and subcommittees held by each organization. The knowledge index ranged from zero to eleven, and was a summation of the elements outlined in the policy knowledge column in Appendix A; one point given if the knowledge was held in the organization and zero if not. Similarly, the skill index ranged from zero to nine, and was created by the number of skills in Appendix A reported by the leader.

This qualitative study likely is influenced by my personal experiences as a participant in an organization similar to the organizations whose leaders participated in the interviews. I am an advocate for more effective SORN policies, but I am not personally influenced by these policies. Interdisciplinary triangulation (Padgett, 1998) was used to minimize the ways in which my personal experiences affected the trustworthiness of this study: Two advisors were recruited during the study based on their discipline (Criminal Justice) and research expertise (Violence against Women) to critically evaluate my potential biases. Overall, my experiences have also worked as a strength for the study, as my participation as a researcher in a similar organization has lent me greater access to this population, and moreover has contributed to a depth of knowledge of the multifaceted issues of SORN policies and the anti-SORN movement.

RESULTS

In the course of my analysis, it became evident that there are two types of anti-SORN SMOs: reactive and proactive organizations. These two groups of organizations were not created a priori; however, based on policy outcomes, I divided the organizations into these two groups. Three of the 19 organizations that participated in the study had not successfully achieved a policy outcome; therefore, I discuss only the results of the remaining 16 organizations. Proactive organizations presented their most successful policy outcome as being on the offense by working to introduce legislation that reduces the harms of registration for registrants and their family members. This type was made up of eight total organizations, five whose leaders reported policy development as their most successful outcome, one organization reporting a policy adoption, and two reporting a substantial policy amendment. Reactive organizations presented their most successful policy outcome as being on the defense by reacting to the policies introduced by state-level policymakers. This grouping is comprised of eight total groups; seven leaders noted that blocking a bill was their most successful outcome, and one leader reported obtaining a minor policy amendment. Based on these categorizations, there were eight proactive and eight reactive organizations (see Table 1).

Organizational Emergence

History. Regardless of the reactive or proactive designation, the majority of the organizations (14 of 16) were started by a registrant or a registrant's family member, most often a mother, daughter, or wife of someone on the registry. One leader from a reactive organization told a story of how she started the organization in her state:

> My husband and I were forced to move from our home that we have lived in, owned and lived in for over 10 years, because of retroactive application of residency restrictions. We didn't handle it real well ...

TABLE 1 Outcome Achieved, Resources & Tactics of Proactive & Reactive Organizations

	All SORN SMOs (*N* = 16)	Proactive (*N* = 8)	Reactive (*N* = 8)
Policy Outcome Achieved			
Block	**7**	0	7
Amend	**3**	2	1
Develop	**5**	5	0
Adopt	**1**	1	0
Resources			
Formalized Structure Index (0–18)	**7.6**	8.5	6.5
Operating Budget	**5**	3	2
Average Number of Volunteers	**9**	10	8
Average Number of Active Members	**45**	45	45
Average Number of Total Members	**186**	181	192
At least 1 Professional Member	**14**	8	6
Profession Types:			
Legal	**12**	8	5
Treatment Provider	**11**	5	6
Researcher	**7**	5	2
Victim's Rights Group	**5**	3	2
Parole/Police	**4**	1	3
Clergy	**2**	1	1
Business	**2**	0	2
Knowledge Index (0–11)	**8.7***	8.4*	9.0
Skill Index (0–9)	**7.3***	7.1*	7.5
Tactics			
Average Number of Tactics Used (0–7)	**2.8**	2.9	2.6
Number that Adapted to the Political Environment	**6**	3	3
Number that used a Political Opportunity	**10**	5	5
Type of Opportunity:			
State Legislature	**5**	2	3
Media Story	**4**	2	2
Court Case	**2**	2	0

*Index could not be calculated for one organization

> We just wanted to deny the whole sex offender registry. He filled out paperwork, nobody talked about it, and all of a sudden this came up. And at that point, I just had enough . . . . When we were forced to move, that punished me and our children because that was our home, too. So really our only choices at that point were to have him not live with us, which punishes us, or move from a home that was ours. And at that point, I really felt it had gone too far because I was being punished for something he had done 25 years ago. At that point I'd had enough.

Almost all of the leaders stated that sex offender management policies have caused harm to registrants and their family members. Moreover, it was these consequences that prompted their participation in the anti-SORN SMO.

Structure. The length of operation for participating anti-SORN SMOs ranged from four months to six years, with the majority operating for five years. Proactive organizations were found to be more formalized on the formalization index (8.5) than reactive organizations (6.5) (see Table 1). Anti-SORN SMOs were determined to have a formalized organizational structure when they reported carrying out tasks such as incorporating the organization with the Internal Revenue Service, building a hierarchy within the organization to streamline decision making, delegating tasks to members to achieve more efficiency and less duplication, and documenting the work of the SMO. While some organizations built formalized structures and processes to bring legitimacy into the political arena, some leaders reported that they did not want their organizations to be formalized to the extent that funding is required for sustainability. One reactive organization leader stated:

> Some organizations I've seen have great goals and aspirations and serve their community, and then they start becoming more and more professional, more and more expensive, and they begin to make commitments: office space and professional staff. And soon they spend all their time fundraising and don't have any time to commit to their constituents. So that's the last thing I want to do, is become that financially burdensome . . . If we could just keep it to printing and mailing and everybody's responsible for getting to where they need to get on their own. I know that sounds like an ad-hoc kind of local organization, but I just dread the thought of making that step to a professional, expensive organization. If you're working for crippled children or for pets or whatever, you can engender support from the community financially, but if you're working with sex offenders, no organization is going to support you with grants.

There is a legitimate concern of the burden of becoming too formalized; however, it is important to note that more of the proactive organizations adopted an infrastructure that was likely to increase their impact with politicians in the political arena.

Resources. Proactive organizations were found to have more resources than reactive organizations (see Table 1). Overall, five organizations had a current operating budget: three proactive organizations and two reactive. The three proactive organizations had budgets between $1,200 and $20,000; reactive organizations were both $2,500. All five organizations received their income from donations, and the three proactive organizations also received income from membership dues.

One of the most important resources of any SMO is the membership, who work to implement the tactics used to impact policy. Leaders were asked about three types of members: those that run the organization as volunteers, the active members of the organization who participate in the strategies toward achieving the organization's policy goals (active members), and the number of individuals who belong to the organization as indicated by being on an e-mail list or receiving the organization's materials (total members). Proactive and reactive organizations were similar in membership: proactive reported an average of 10 volunteers and reactive had eight; both had an average of 45 active members; total membership averaged 181 for proactive organizations and 192 for reactive.

Although registrants and their family members are the most likely to be negatively affected by sex offender laws, the stigma that is associated with this population is likely to delegitimize the organization. One way to build legitimacy is to have individuals who are not personally affected by SORN policies educate legislators on the issues. Most often, this is achieved by members who have professional expertise related to registered sex offenders. Table 1 includes the findings of professional membership, with a few key differences when comparing proactive and reactive organizations. All proactive organizations and six reactive organizations included at least one professional member. All proactive organizations had legal representation, compared to five reactive organizations. More proactive organizations reported having a researcher in the organization (five, compared to two in reactive organizations). More reactive organizations reported that they had police/parole and business members. Similar numbers were reported for treatment providers, victim's rights groups, and clergy (see Table 1). Building on these professional members is likely to increase the effectiveness of these organizations in their use of tactics and at achieving a policy outcome.

SORN knowledge. Surprisingly, in the analysis of proactive and reactive organizations, members of proactive organizations on average had less SORN policy knowledge (8.4, compared to 9.0 for reactive organizations, see Table 1). All proactive and reactive organizations reported knowledge related to the reasons that SORN laws were created, the assumptions that underlie these policies, the effectiveness that these policies have in reaching their intended goals, and the impact that the policies have on registrants. Six reactive and three proactive leaders reported a deficit in knowledge that notes the impact that these policies have on victims of sexual violence. Another deficit of knowledge is in regard to having an alternative policy ready to present to legislators, with only four proactive organizations and six reactive organizations having this at their disposal. Of organizations that have an alternative policy, all of the proactive organizations have information about the outcomes of the alternative policy, whereas only three of the six reactive organizations know the outcomes. Only five organizations were able to present the tradeoffs between the current SORN policies and the alternative policy they proposed: two proactive and three reactive. Regarding alternative policies, one reactive leader stated the following:

> We had some . . . I think that's sort of a lacking area. Cause I don't think it's as simple as some people say . . . I think public education needs to play a huge part of developing what that [alternative policies] would look like . . . Also, setting up ways for people who need treatment so that

> they can self-report needing treatment. The way a person self-reports using illegal drugs . . . They can report to rehab centers and it doesn't necessarily prevent them from getting any kind of punishment but it is mitigated by it.

As with most anti-SORN SMOs with alternative policies, this leader supported public education and treatment as an alternative policy to reduce sexual violence. It seems counterintuitive that the proactive organizations reported less policy knowledge than the reactive organizations. It may be that the most compelling pieces of SORN policy knowledge that the proactive organizations use are in the areas most important to policymakers and the public. The areas of knowledge reported more often by reactive organizations may not influence arguments with policymakers or the public.

Advocacy skills. Reactive organizations reported more types of advocacy skills (7.5 on skill index) than proactive organizations (7.1). Almost all of the anti-SORN SMO leaders in both proactive and reactive organizations noted that someone in the organization had the necessary skills to analyze policy or legislation, write and deliver a presentation, build relationships with policymakers and government bureaucrats, and someone who was able to give a media interview. However, only half of the leaders, three proactive and four reactive, believed that someone in their organization was able to work from inside the system, meaning that they could navigate the political environment. This lack of working inside the system most likely stems from the number of years anti-SORN SMOs have been operating and also the inability of politicians to be open to hearing their position. When one proactive leader was asked about working inside the system, she analogized, "I'm trying, but boy, sometimes it feels like we're David and they're the Goliath." Many have not been offered the opportunity to work with legislators on this issue. Contrary to what would be expected, it was found that proactive organizations reported fewer advocacy skills. It is surmised that while they may not have a broad range of skills, they may be more adept at the skills they do have, such as building relationships with elected officials.

Tactics

Overall, anti-SORN SMOs reported using tactics that allow the organization and the politicians who support them to keep a low profile. Lobbying and policymaker education, research and policy analysis, and membership mobilization were the dominant tactics. One proactive leader described lobbying and policymaker education:

> So it's meeting with the individuals on a particular committee and educating them one by one, giving them tools and facts, and approaching it from, "Look, my purpose here is to give you the tools you need to have

to make an informed decision so that you don't fall prey to the misinformation, public panic and hysteria, but you can base your decisions on fact." And you know, we always ask [legislators] the question, "Tell me how I can help you to educate your constituents, so that you can do the right thing."

Research and policy analysis were explicitly or implicitly noted as useful in all of the achieved policy outcomes by all but two of the organizations. Since all of the organizations are working on changing policy, they must learn how to read current legislation and any new bills that are focused on registrants. The two remaining proactive anti-SORN SMOs relied heavily on a constitutional rights argument, in place of data that shows SORN is an ineffective policy. Proactive organizations used a wider variety of tactics and were more likely to use network and coalition building and media interviews. Conversely, more reactive organizations used testimony and research and policy analysis. Reactive anti-SORN SMOs used grassroots organizing and mobilization and electronic outreach when a quick response was needed from the membership, generally to attend a hearing on short notice.

To date, tactics that garner public attention and legal advocacy or litigation have not been used by anti-SORN SMOs to achieve their most successful policy outcome. Tactics used to garner public attention include public and voter education, polling the public, endorsement of political candidates, and rallies or marches. Many of the leaders suggested that the media is highly stigmatizing to anti-SORN SMOs. As such, only three, two from proactive organizations and one from a reactive organization, reported approaching the media to do a story on their advocacy efforts. One reactive leader suggested that the high level of stigmatization toward registrants is because of the media: "Primarily, that's [stigma] due to how the media presents these issues and the lack of a balanced presentation of the facts relating to sex offenders."

Adapting to the political environment. Political opportunity theory argues that SMOs will adapt to the environment by changing the tactics they use to achieve their outcome (Kriesi, 2007). Only six leaders (three proactive and three reactive organizations) discussed cases in which the organization had changed tactics. One proactive and one reactive leader suggested that their organizations changed the way they testify in committee hearings by reducing the number of individuals who testify and separating the key points that need to be covered. The reactive leader stated, "It's hard though, starting out as a group like this and growing. Getting to know what you should and shouldn't do and how to say things appropriately. It takes a while." One proactive organization changed the focus of one of its policies after receiving pertinent information from political insiders. This leader said, "We got some very strong negative feedback in terms of going forward with [the bill] from both the legislature and from some of the lawyers we worked with and someone who really tried to help us." This organization was advised to take up this particular bill at a time in the political process when it would be more likely to be passed by the legislature.

After one organization was ignored by policymakers, its members decided that, in the future, they are changing their dominant tactic from legislative change to legal advocacy and litigation. The leader of this proactive organization said:

> They basically disrespected us last spring at the legislature by killing our bill unanimously in committee and not listening to us. Our answer to that is, "OK, if you won't listen to us we'll do it ourselves" . . . They better take us seriously if we raise $10,000 for litigation that takes everybody off the registry convicted prior to 2002. That will get attention.

One reactive leader discussed a situation in which his group changed the particulars of a policy that they wanted to amend once they realized that a new bill created room for negotiation with the state legislature. He stated:

> We really wanted to address our other issues, but we had to focus on this because they were moving on this [policy], so it forced us to put our attention on this [policy], and diverted our attention away from the things we really wanted to see changed in the law . . . . So our energy was focused more on what we could do within the law . . . . It gave us an opportunity to get changes in there that might have taken longer to get otherwise.

Another reactive leader said that her group changed the way they advocate when her organization realized that juveniles and youthful registrants garner more sympathy from policymakers. She commented:

> In a sense, we sort of use that [young registrants] to help open the door for other ones, because when they recognize that these kinds of individuals are labeled and yet they're low risk for re-offense, then that's when it sort of opens the door to talk about risk assessment and [who] really is the kind of person you'd have register.

Political opportunities. Leaders were asked about any opportunities that arose in the legislature, the media, or the courts that they used to help persuade a policymaker to side with their organization's successful policy outcome. Five proactive and five reactive organizations reported one or more opportunities. Two proactive and three reactive leaders noted that they used an opportunity in the state legislature; two proactive and two reactive organizations used a story found in the media related to sexual crimes or registration; and two proactive organizations used a court case. When one anti-SORN SMO was working to develop a bill that would ban residency restrictions, they referred to a district court decision that stated such restrictions are unconstitutional. The proactive organization's leader stated, "We capitalized on the court decision to say, 'You have an unconstitutional law. What are you going to do about it? You took an oath to uphold the constitution of [state name].'" The other proactive organization used an appellate court case that found registration to be cruel and unusual punishment for cases involving consensual sexual acts prosecuted under statutory rape laws. This led to their successful quest to remove similar laws altogether from state legislation.

The leader of the proactive organization above also used a story that was portrayed in the media to secure and expand public support. This organization worked with individuals in the media to present a sympathetic consensual statutory rape case that showed the collateral consequences of registration for young offenders. The leader would discuss the news story when she met with legislators. A similar situation was reported by a reactive organization that used a sympathetic case in the media to block a bill. Another proactive leader described the use of a different type of media portrayal. This organization had developed a policy requiring the removal of some offenses from public registration. At that time, there was a national news story about university athletes who were falsely accused of rape. This leader added, "I believe it helped because the politicians, especially the one I was working with, saw how girls and young ladies can lie." The final reactive organization that used the media as an opportunity happened when a state was working to develop residency restrictions. There were news reports regarding concerns that the policy would remove sex offenders from their homes, thus making them homeless.

Five organizations noted that they used an opportunity in the legislature to their advantage when achieving a policy outcome. One proactive and one reactive leader explicitly stated that they used their states' budgetary issues to their advantage. One proactive and one reactive organization used their established rapport with a particular political party to advance their policy goal. One proactive leader explained that policymakers share information among themselves, especially when they work on the same committees. This leader described a situation in which the anti-SORN SMO gained support from an unlikely policymaker when another policymaker with whom the organization already had ties persuaded his colleague to support an amendment to a punitive SORN policy. A reactive leader noted that he gained the support of two legislators who controlled the bills that would be heard in a committee. The respondent stated, "They [the two legislators] worked very closely to manipulate the agenda to eliminate the [bill]". In this situation, time ran out for the introduction of new bills, which meant that the bill would be postponed until the next legislative session. The political process/opportunities theories suggest that policy change occurs when organizations use opportunities to their advantage. To date, both proactive and reactive anti-SORN SMOs have used the opportunities available to them to persuade legislators to make changes to SORN policy.

DISCUSSION

This study presents the first rigorous investigation of social movement organizations that are attempting to change SORN policies. In this study I ask, What organizational factors, including structure, resources, knowledge, and skill, are associated with anti-SORN SMOs reporting successful achievement of a policy outcome? Anti-SORN SMOs have been operating for a relatively short time and are most often led by a family member of a registrant or registrants themselves. This reveals that this social movement is relatively new and is deeply personal to the individuals within the organizations. Anti-SORN SMOs have very few material resources, with only five participating organizations reporting an operating budget. With lower levels of material resources than other social movements, one might conclude that anti-SORN SMOs are destined for failure; however, the type of movement may have a greater impact on the longevity and success of anti-SORN SMOs (Kriesi, 1996). These organizations are part of an identity-driven movement, which suggests a high level of commitment on the part of the membership that will sustain the group despite having lower resource levels than other movements (Kriesi, 1996).

Proactive organizations are more formalized and have more resources compared to reactive organizations. An interesting finding is that, of the organizations that had an operating budget, only the proactive organizations were collecting membership dues. An increased level of formalization and more resources of proactive organizations is likely because these organizations have different motivations than reactive organizations, by taking charge of their own destiny to make things better, as opposed to only stopping things from getting worse (i.e., blocking policies).

The findings of this study show that there is a consistently reported issue of policymakers and the media not taking these organizations seriously, due to the target population of this movement. Building a list of professional allies, who are not personally affected by this issue, will likely increase anti-SORN SMO legitimacy. This, in turn, will assist anti-SORN SMOs in gaining access to the political environment. Oftentimes, social workers with expertise in sex offender treatment acted as professional members in these organizations. Furthermore, social workers who belonged to victim rights organizations sat down with these anti-SORN SMOs to find areas where they could work together on policy changes. Thus, there are key professional roles that social workers play within these advocacy organizations that help raise awareness and bring legitimacy to the claims made by registrants and their family members.

The findings of this study show differences in the types of professional members within proactive and reactive organizations. First, every proactive organization had at least one professional member, while two reactive organizations did not have any professional members. Second, more proactive organizations reported having a legal professional and a researcher in their organization, whereas more reactive organizations reported having parole or probation and business professional members. A common skill deficit reported by over half of the organizations (three proactive and four reactive) was that there were no members in the organization that were able to work from inside the system. This is likely because policymakers view these organizations as lacking legitimacy. Thus, finding ways to build relationships in the system is a key task for anti-SORN SMOs, as suggested in a study of state legislator's perspectives on effective interest groups (Teater, 2009). Teater (2009) suggests that relationship building is a process whereby legislators determine if individuals from the interest group are credible, in that they keep the promises they make to the legislator; they personalize the information they offer to legislators by the medium and content of their communications; and they have a consistent and knowledgeable presence at the state capital. Extending these criteria to all types of advocacy groups is important, but these concepts are critical for advocacy groups that are focused on stigmatized and marginalized populations.

An important finding is that the organizational knowledge needed to be effective in the political environment is the result of a lack of an alternative policy proposal. Anti-SORN SMOs should be ready with an alternative policy proposal that addresses the issues with current policies and discusses the projected outcomes from the new proposal, with discussion of the tradeoffs between the two policies. Anti-SORN SMOs may be more likely to achieve greater outcomes if the proposal is ready to go when a political opportunity arises (Kingdon, 2003; Teater, 2009). More reactive organizations reported having an alternative policy; however, only half were able to both present the predicted outcomes of the alternative policy and discuss the tradeoffs between SORN and the alternative policy. Proactive organizations that had an alternative policy also had projected outcomes of this policy ready, and all but one could discuss the tradeoffs.

This study also asked, How do these organizational factors, along with the political environment, shape the strategy and tactics used to achieve a policy outcome? Anti-SORN SMOs are likely to use tactics that do not bring public attention to this issue. Due to the stigma that is associated with this population and the way the media perpetuates moral panic regarding sex offenders, these organizations are cautious when using the media to gain public support. This tactic may lead to a backlash. Generally, this tactic has been used to create political opportunities for other social movements

(Gamson & Meyer, 1996); however, many anti-SORN SMOs believe that the media has created hysteria about sex offenders and continues to perpetuate misinformation (Leon, 2011). Therefore, some anti-SORN SMOs do not see the media as a way to open up political opportunities. Proactive organizations used the media, along with networking and coalition building more than reactive organizations. Reactive organizations were more likely to use research and policy analysis and testimony. It is not surprising that the organizations that reported their most successful policy outcome as blocking a policy would use testimony and research and policy analysis tactics most frequently. Testimony is generally the most common way to block a policy in a committee hearing.

Adaptation to the political environment and taking advantage of opportunities are crucial to achieving a successful policy outcome. Six organizations (three proactive and three reactive) reported changes in tactics used to achieve the organization's goals. Therefore, as a whole, these organizations are relatively inflexible in adapting to the state's political environment. This may be so because the organizations have been operating for a short time, and thus have had little time to adapt their tactics. Anti-SORN SMOs took advantage of three opportunities in conjunction with their achieved policy outcome: court cases related to SORN policies that were likely to influence new legislation; media portrayals of consequences for registered offenders; and events in the state's legislature. Tarrow (1996) suggests three elements that open opportunities in the policy environment: creating an opening in the environment, using influential allies, and dividing elites in the environment. Anti-SORN SMO leaders mentioned that an opening in the environment and the use of influential allies (professionals and individual policymakers) have created opportunities for engagement in the political environment; however, none reported the division of elites.

In sum, proactive organizations were more formalized, more likely to collect membership dues, and more likely to have legal and research professional members. Furthermore, more proactive organizations reported the use of media interviews and networking and coalition building as tactics toward their most successful policy outcome and they were more likely to use court rulings to persuade politicians to change SORN policy. For stigmatized advocacy organizations that want to develop and create beneficial policies, these tactics and strategies will be most useful. Reactive organizations were more likely to have police/parole or business professional members, and were more likely to use research and policy analysis and testimony as the tactics used to achieve their most successful policy outcome. In addition, reactive organizations were more likely to use opportunities in the state's legislature to achieve their most successful policy outcome. Thus, when attempting to block policies that harm stigmatized populations, these are the most useful tactics and strategies.

In the future, studies should include additional sources of organizational information to enhance our understanding of these organizations and their influence on state-level policy (for example, meeting minutes of the members and board of directors, by-laws, newsletters, or mass e-mails sent to the membership). State-level policymakers could also be interviewed to determine the influence that these organizations have on their decision making for SORN legislation (see Teater, 2009). Multiple voices within each organization should be surveyed for their perceptions related to resources, tactics, and strategies. Finally, the differences found between the proactive and reactive organizations should be investigated more intensely in the future in order to discern which resources and tactics have the greatest influence on successful policy strategies. For example, an interesting finding of this study was that reactive organizations reported a broader range of SORN policy knowledge. Thus, a follow up study is needed that investigates the specific areas of knowledge that is most influential in creating policy change.

REFERENCES

Buechler, S. (1995). Social movement theories. *The Sociological Quarterly, 36*(3), 441–464.

Burgess, A., & Holstrom, L. (1974). *Rape: Crisis and recovery*. Bowie, MD: Brady.

Clark, M. (2012). States struggle with national sex offender law. *Stateline: State policy & politics*, Thursday, January 5, 2012. Retrieved from http://www.stateline.org/live/details/story?contentId=622764.

Comartin, E., Kernsmith, P., & Miles, B. (2010). Family experiences of young adult sex offender registration. *Journal of Child Sexual Abuse, 19*(2), 204–225.

Council on Social Work Education [CSWE]. (2008). Educational policy and accreditation standards. Retrieved from http://www.cswe.org/Accreditation/2008EPASDescription.aspx.

Cresswell, J., & Miller, D. (2000). Determining validity in qualitative inquiry. *Theory into Practice, 39*(3), 124–130.

Davis, G., McAdam, D., Scott, W., & Zald, M. (2006). *Social movement and organization theory*. New York, NY: Cambridge University Press.

Edwards, B., & McCarthy, J. (2007). Resources and social movement mobilization. In D. Snow, S. Soule, & H. Kriesi (Eds.), *The Blackwell companion to social movements* (pp. 116–152). London, England: Blackwell.

Finn, P. (1997). *Sex offender community notification*. Washington, DC: U.S. Department of Justice: Office of Justice Programs.

Gamson, J., & Meyer, D. (1996). Framing political opportunity. In D. McAdam, J. McCarthy, & M. Zald (Eds.), *Comparative perspectives on social movements: Political opportunities, mobilizing structures, and cultural framings* (pp. 275–290). New York, NY: Cambridge University Press.

Geiger, B. (2006). The case for treating ex-offenders as a suspect class. *California Law Review, 94*(4), 1191–1242.

Glaser, B., & Strauss, A. (1967). *The discovery of grounded theory: Strategies for qualitative research*. Chicago, IL: Aldine.

Grubesic, T., Mack, E., & Murray, A. (2007). Geographic exclusion: Spatial analysis for evaluating the implications of Megan's law. *Social Science Computer Review, 25*, 143–162.

Harvard Family Research Project (HFRP). (2009). A user's guide to advocacy evaluation planning. Retrieved from http://www.hfrp.org/evaluation/publications-resources/a-user-s-guide-to-advocacy-evaluation-planning.

Hoefer, R. (2006). *Advocacy practice in social justice*. Chicago, IL: Lyceum Books, Inc.

Human Rights Watch. (2007). *No easy answer: Sex offender laws in the U.S.* Retrieved from http://www.hrw.org/reports/2007/us0907.

Jenkins, P. (1998). *Moral panic: Changing concepts of the child molester in modern America*. New Haven, CT: Yale University Press.

Kingdon, J. (2003). *Agendas, alternatives, and public policies* (2nd ed.) New York, NY: Addison-Wesley Educational Publishers, Inc.

Kriesi, H. (1996). The organizational structure of new social movements in a political context. In D. McAdam, J. McCarthy, & M. Zald (Eds.), *Comparative perspectives on social movements: Political opportunities, mobilizing structures, and cultural framings* (pp. 152–184). New York, NY: Cambridge University Press.

Kriesi, H. (2007). Political context and opportunity. In D. Snow, S. Soule, & H. Kriesi (Eds.), *The Blackwell companion to social movements* (pp. 67–90). Malden, MA: Blackwell Publishing Ltd.

Leon, C. (2011). *Sex fiends, perverts, and pedophiles: Understanding sex crime policy in America*. New York, NY: New York University Press.

Levenson, J. (2008). Collateral consequences of sex offender residence restrictions. *Criminal Justice Studies, 21*(2), 153–166.

Levenson, J., D'Amora, D., & Hern, A. (2007). Megan's law and its impact on community re-entry of sex offenders. *Behavioral Sciences and the Law, 25*, 587–602.

Levenson, J., & Tewksbury, R. (2009). Collateral damage: Family members of registered sex offenders. *American Journal of Criminal Justice, 34*(1/2), 54–68.

Lewis, C. (1996). The Jacob Wetterling Crimes Against Children and Sexually Violent Offender Registration Act: An unconstitutional deprivation of the right to privacy and substantive due process. *Harvard Civil Rights-Civil Liberties Law Review, 31*(1), 89–118.

Logan, W. (2009). *Knowledge as power: Criminal registration and community notification laws in America*. Stanford, CA: Stanford Law Books.

Mancini, C., & Mears, D. (2013). U.S. Supreme Court decisions and sex offender legislation: Evidence of evidence-based policy? *Journal of Criminal Law and Criminology, 103*(4), 1115–1153.

McAdam, D. (1994). Conceptual origins, current problems, future directions. In D. McAdam, J. McCarthy, & M. Zald (Eds.), *Comparative perspectives on social movements: Political opportunities, mobilizing structures, and cultural framings*, (pp. 23–40). New York, NY: Cambridge University Press.

McAdam, D., & Scott, R. (2005). Organizations and movements. In G. Davis, D. McAdam, R. Scott, & M. Zald (Eds.), *Social movements and organizational theory*, (pp. 4–40). Cambridge, UK: Cambridge University Press.

McCarthy, J. (1996). Constraints and opportunities in adopting, adapting and inventing. In, D. McAdam, J. McCarthy, & M. Zald (Eds.), *Comparative perspectives on social movements: Political opportunity, mobilizing structures, and cultural framings*, (pp. 141–151). New York, NY: Cambridge University Press.

McPhail, C. (1991). *The myth of the madding crowd*. New York, NY: Aldine de Gruyter.

National Association of Social Workers [NASW]. (2008). Code of Ethics. Washington, DC: National Association of Social Workers.

National Center for Missing and Exploited Children. (2011). Map of registered sex offenders in the United States. Retrieved from http://www.missingkids.com/en_US/documents/sex-offender-map.pdf

National Conference of State Legislatures. (2012). Adam Walsh Child Protection and Safety Act: Compliance news. Retrieved from http://www.ncsl.org/issues-research/justice/adam-walsh-child-protection-and-safety-act.aspx

Newman, M. (2012). Maps of the 2008 US presidential election results. Department of Physics and Center for the Study of Complex Systems, University of Michigan. Retrieved from http://www-personal.umich.edu/~mejn/election/2008/

Office of Sex Offender Sentencing, Monitoring, Apprehending, Registering, and Tracking. (2011). Newsroom: Jurisdictions that have substantially implemented SORNA. Retrieved from http://www.ojp.usdoj.gov/smart/newsroom.htm

Padgett, D. (1998). *Qualitative methods in social work research*. Thousand Oaks, CA: Sage.

Reisman, J., Gienapp, A., & Stachowiak, S. (2007). A guide to measuring advocacy and policy. Retrieved from http://www.aecf.org/KnowledgeCenter/Publications.aspx?pubguid={4977C910-1A39-44BD-A106-1FC8D81EB792}

Rothenberg, L. (1992). *Linking citizens to government: Interest group politics at common cause*. Cambridge, UK: Cambridge University Press.

Rubin, A., & Babbie, E. (2010). *Essential research methods for social work* (2nd ed.). Belmont, CA: Brooks/Cole, Cengage Learning.

Saunders, E. (1988). A comparative study of attitudes toward child sexual abuse among social work and judicial system professionals. *Child Abuse & Neglect*, *12*, 83–90.

Smith v. Doe, 538 U.S. 84 (2003).

State v. Williams, 952 N.E.2d 1108, 1112 (Ohio 2011).

Strauss, A., & Corbin, J. (1990). *Basics of qualitative research: Grounded theory procedures and techniques*. Newbury Park, CA: Sage.

Tarrow, S. (1996). States and opportunities: The political structuring of social movements. In D. McAdam, J. McCarthy, & M. Zald (Eds.), *Comparative perspectives on social movements: Political opportunities, mobilizing structures, and cultural framings* (pp. 41–61). New York, NY: Cambridge University Press.

Teater, B. (2009). Influencing state legislators: A framework for developing effective social work interest groups. *Journal of Policy Practice*, *8*, 69–86.

Terry, K., & Ackerman, A. (2009). A brief history of major sex offender laws. In R. Wright (Ed.), *Sex offender laws: Failed policies, new directions*, (pp. 65–98). New York, NY: Springer Publishing Company.

Tewksbury, R. (2005). Collateral consequences of sex offender registration. *Journal of Contemporary Criminal Justice*, *21*(1), 67–81.

Tewksbury, R., Jennings, W., & Zgoba, K. (2012). *Final report on sex offenders: Recidivism and collateral consequences* (United States Department of Justice, report #238060. Retrieved from https://www.ncjrs.gov/App/AbstractDB/AbstractDBDetails.aspx?id=260103

Tewksbury, R., & Lees, M. (2006). Perceptions of sex offender registration: Collateral consequences and community experiences. *Sociological Spectrum, 26*(3), 309–334.

Tilly, C., & Rule, J. (1965). *Measuring political upheaval*. Princeton, NJ: Center for International Studies, Princeton University.

U.S. Census Bureau. (2010). Interactive population map. Retrieved from http://2010.census.gov/2010census/popmap/

U.S. Census Bureau. (2011). Census regions and divisions of the United States. U.S. Department of Commerce and Economic Statistics Administration: Geography Department. Retrieved from http://www.census.gov/geo/www/2010census/gtc/gtc_census_divreg.html

U.S. Census Bureau. (2012). Households and families: 2010. Retrieved from http://www.census.gov/prod/cen2010/briefs/c2010br-14.pdf

Van Horn, C., Baumer, D., & Gromley, W. (2001). *Politics and public policy* (3rd ed.). Washington, DC: CQ Press.

Whittier, N. (2009). *The politics of child sexual abuse: Emotion, social movements, and the state*. New York, NY: Oxford University Press.

Zald, M., & Ash, R. (1966). Social movement organizations: Growth, decay and change. *Social Forces, 44*, 327–340.

APPENDIX A. KNOWLEDGE ABOUT SORN POLICIES & ADVOCACY SKILLS LISTS

Knowledge	Skills
1. The reasons that Sex Offender Registration and Community Notification (SORN) policies were created.	1. Analyzing legislation or policy.
2. The assumptions about sex offenders that underlie SORN policies.	2. Prepare a briefing note or position paper.
3. Studies or statistics about the effectiveness or ineffectiveness of current policies.	3. Writing and delivering a presentation.
4. Studies or statistics related to the impact that SORN policies have on victims of sexual violence.	4. Building relationships with political decision makers.
5. Studies or statistics related to the impact that SORN policies have on registered sex offenders.	5. Persuasion Skills.
6. Studies or statistics related to the impact that SORN policies have on the community at-large.	6. Negotiation skills.
7. Studies or statistics of the costs involved in implementing SORN policies at the state level.	7. Working from inside the system.
8. Major federal or state Supreme Court decisions related to SORN policies.	8. Writing and using a press release.
9. Alternative courses of action that might be taken to solve the issue of sexual violence.	9. Carrying out a media interview.
10. Projected outcomes from the alternative courses of action mentioned above.	
11. Knowledge of the tradeoffs between current SORN policies and the alternative policies to solve the problem.	

APPENDIX B. POLICY OUTCOMES LIST

Policy Outcome	Definition
1. Policy Blocking	1. Successful opposition to a policy proposal. Member(s) of the organization work with legislators to block bills that the organization believes will decrease the quality of life for registered sex offenders.
2. Placement on the Policy Agenda	2. The appearance of an issue or policy proposal on the list of issues that policymakers give serious attention.
3. Policy Amendment	3. The process of altering or adding text to a policy proposal.
4. Policy Development	4. Developing a specific policy solution for the issue or problem being addressed. Creating a new policy or policy guidelines.
5. Policy Adoption	5. Successful passing of a policy proposal through an ordinance, ballot measure, legislation, or legal agreement.
6. Policy Implementation	6. Proper implementation of a policy, along with the funding, resources, or quality assurance to ensure it.
7. Policy Monitoring and Evaluation	7. Tracking a policy to ensure it is implemented properly and achieves its intended impacts.
8. Policy Maintenance	8. Preventing cuts or other negative changes to a policy.

NASW Involvement in Legislative Advocacy

DAVID BEIMERS
Minnesota State University, Mankato, Minnesota, USA

NASW serves as the professional association for social workers, yet little is known about how NASW chapters engage social workers and social work students in policy practice. This article presents the results of a survey of 40 NASW state chapters, describing how NASW engages social workers in legislative advocacy, the role of legislative advocacy days, and the involvement of social work students in NASW advocacy efforts. Findings indicate state chapters are very involved in policy practice and legislative advocacy days appear to be one prominent vehicle in engaging members and social work students in legislative advocacy.

This study examines the role of state chapters of the National Association of Social Workers (NASW) in preparing social work students and professionals to be policy practitioners. Much has been written over the past two decades about the political activity of social workers (Ezell, 1993; Hamilton & Fauri, 2001; Ritter, 2007; Ritter, 2008; Rocha, Poe, & Thomas, 2010; Rome & Hoechstetter, 2010), as well as how social work educators prepare future social workers to engage in policy practice (Anderson & Harris, 2005; Bernklau Halvor, 2012; DeRigne, Rosenwald, & Naranjo, 2014; Fitzgerald & McNutt, 1999; Manalo, 2004; Powell & Causby, 1994; Rocha, 2000). As the preeminent member organization associated with the social work profession, NASW is well positioned to serve as a political voice for social workers. Through statewide conferences and legislative advocacy days, NASW has a key role in developing and advancing the profession. As a member organization, NASW also has a commitment to social work values, which includes advocating for social and economic justice. Despite this key role, there have been few studies that have examined NASW's role in facilitating advocacy among social work professionals (Hartnett, Harding, & Scanlon, 2005; Salcido & Seck, 1992; Scanlon, Hartnett, & Harding, 2006) or developing advocacy skills in students (Kilbane, Pryce, & Hong, 2013). Currently, no studies have examined the role of legislative advocacy days as a part of NASW chapter activities.

NASW is the largest membership organization of professional social workers in the world, with more than 132,000 members in 55 chapters. Part of the mission of the NASW, as stated on the organization's website, is to "advance sound social policies" (www.socialworkers.org/nasw). NASW does facilitate political action at the federal level through several initiatives. Some of these initiatives focus on educational and professional issues, such as the Action Network for Social Work Education and Research (ANSWER), which advocates on behalf of social work education, training and research, and the Social Work Reinvestment Initiative. NASW also facilitates advocacy at the national level on federal legislation affecting both social workers and the populations that social workers serve. This is accomplished through developing policy positions, using e-mail listserv advocacy, and hosting a Political Action for Candidate Election (PACE) committee, which endorses and financially supports candidates who have political views that are aligned with NASW.

Purpose

The purpose of this study is to better understand ways in which state chapters of NASW are involving members and students in advocacy. Policy practice has a central role in the professional responsibilities of social workers. The Council on Social Work Education (CSWE) has clearly identified policy practice as a core competency to be attained as a part of social work education (CSWE, 2012). Furthermore, the NASW Code of Ethics (2008) identifies advocating for policy change as an ethical responsibility (6.04). Given this focus, it makes sense that NASW chapters would engage in fulfilling this professional expectation. However, it is currently unknown how NASW chapters involve social work professionals and students in developing or applying policy practice skills. This study has three main research questions: (1) how do local chapters of NASW engage social work students in advocacy efforts; (2) how do local chapters of NASW engage social work professionals in advocacy efforts; and (3) what role do legislative advocacy days serve in the advocacy efforts of NASW chapters?

LITERATURE REVIEW

Much of the literature on the legislative advocacy of social workers has focused on two areas; the extent to which professional social workers are engaged in advocacy and how social work programs train social work students to engage in policy practice. Few studies have explored the role of NASW chapters in engaging social workers and social work students in advocacy. This literature review will begin by reviewing (1) what we know about social workers engaging in advocacy, then (2) how social work programs prepare students to be advocates, (3) addressing the literature on social service groups and coalitions engaging in advocacy, and finally, (4) NASW chapters engagement in policy practice.

Social Work Engagement in Advocacy

One of the earliest studies of political participation among social workers examined National Association of Social Work (NASW) members in Michigan and found that social workers were more politically active than the general population, but less active than other professionals (Wolk, 1981). Race, social work position, affiliation with a professional association, and higher education have all been found to predict increased political activity among social workers (Ezell, 1993).

More recent studies have documented that professional social workers tend to be more politically engaged than the general public, with as many as 90% of social workers reporting advocacy as a key part of their professional role (Ezell, 2001) and 60% of social workers reporting some contact with government officials (Hamilton & Fauri, 2001). Membership in NASW is one professional factor that has been identified as predicting political participation (Hamilton & Fauri, 2001; Ritter, 2007).

Rome and Hoechstetter found that among NASW members, while the majority voted regularly, stayed informed about news, and monitored legislation, respondents were less involved in organizing or participating in rallies or marches, testifying at hearings, or even contacting legislators (Rome & Hoechstetter, 2010). Efficacy has been found to be a key predictor of participation in political action among social work professionals (Anderson & Harris, 2005; Ezell, 1993; Ritter, 2007, 2008; Weiss, Gal, & Katan, 2006). One common strategy to build this sense of efficacy is through social work education.

Social Work Students and Policy Practice

The development of social work students as competent policy practitioners is now an expectation of all accredited social work programs at the graduate and undergraduate levels (CSWE, 2008). One way that schools of social work have begun to address this perceived inequity is with applied policy practice exercises as part of the social work student's academic experience (Weaver & Nackerud, 2005; Tower & Hash, 2013). The education literature is replete with examples of how social work faculty have provided experiential opportunities as a way for social work students to build advocacy skills (DeRigne, Rosenwald, & Naranjo, 2014). This application of knowledge to practice is consistent with the emphasis on competency-based education.

Research from experiential advocacy courses have found that students are significantly more likely to identify as competent and continue to engage in policy practice after graduation (Manalo, 2004; Rocha, 2000; Tower & Hartnett, 2011). A study that required students to subscribe to an NASW email list and take action on policy items indicated that students were more likely to continue to stay involved following graduation (Tower & Hartnett, 2011). Students involved in an applied exercise called The Advocacy Project reported an increased sense of self-confidence and sense of empowerment, as well as an increased likelihood of continuing to engage in legislative advocacy (Butler & Coleman, 1997). Master of Social Work (MSW) students participating in a political intervention project that paired them with community-based mentors reported that the project, as compared to other course assignments, had the greatest impact on their development of policy intervention skills, perceived capacity to change policy, likelihood of engaging in policy practice in the future, and comfort level in giving opinions on policy issues (Saulnier, 2000). After graduating, 92% reported that they continued to be active in policy practice as part of their social work career (Saulnier, 2000).

Almost all (92%) of the MSW students who were involved in legislative advocacy as part of a policy practice course reported that they were likely to continue to engage in policy practice after the completion of the course, in contrast to a majority indicating they were unlikely to do so prior to the start of the class (Manalo, 2004). A qualitative evaluation of another MSW legislative advocacy project found that it encouraged the students to be more self-confident and skilled as professional social work advocates (Powell & Causby, 1994). In a comparison of two different experiential approaches, undergraduate social work students in both groups reported an increase in knowledge and skill working on social and economic justice issues, as well as an increase in confidence in carrying out policy practice skills in the future (Anderson & Harris, 2005).

As applied policy practice exercises appear to have a positive effect on student learning, efficacy, and intent to advocate in the future, social work educators should look to human service interest groups, including NASW, as potential partners to build advocacy skills in social work students. DeRigne and colleagues (2014) identified a number of models and strategies that incorporate projects with NASW and advocacy days to support student learning and skill development.

Groups and Coalitions

Involvement in human service interest groups can provide a venue for human service professionals, including social workers, to engage in collective action. Interest groups have been found to provide an important source of information to lawmakers, especially at the state level (Jackson-Elmoore, 2005). In a study of four states, Hoefer (2000) found that the most important incentives for participating in interest groups were advocacy of ideas and representing member opinions to government. In regard to the types of strategies that were viewed as important in influencing state policy, respondents reported that working with bureaucracy and working with legislators were most important (Hoefer, 2000), although effective models at the federal level do not necessarily extend to the state level (Hoefer, 2005).

In a qualitative study of state legislators, Teater (2008) identified interest groups as using a process of advice and consultation, where the legislators and interest groups engage in a collaborative relationship that addresses change. Interest group members have specific knowledge and expertise that can be of benefit to decision makers. Still, influencing state policy can be a challenging process and although often social workers have a thorough understanding of limitations of social welfare policy, they may not have the time or resources to affect change. Working through interest groups such as NASW can serve as a vehicle to push for social policy changes in an effective manner (Jackson-Elmoore, 2006).

The Internet is an increasingly common strategy that is used by social work member groups and coalitions to advocate on behalf of social issues. However, some groups have fallen short in their use of the Internet to mobilize and organize members (Edwards & Hoefer, 2010). NASW chapters have been found to be more effective in terms of facilitating communication with lawmakers and providing clear guidance on what actions to take, although with significant room to improve (Edwards & Hoefer, 2010).

The literature reflects that being a part of an organization is an important factor in predicting involvement in advocacy. Groups and organizations can facilitate advocacy by providing a vehicle for involvement and decision-makers report that they value the input of members. A few studies have examined the role of NASW in specific in facilitating advocacy among members.

NASW Chapters

A first look at the political participation of NASW chapters was conducted by Salcido and Seck in 1992. They found that roughly two-thirds of chapters had a political action committee. Areas where chapters were most active involved direct contact with legislators, such as writing letters or calling elected officials (Salcido & Seck, 1992). Chapters were less involved in voter registration efforts and rallies. Similarly, chapter officials reported that they perceived lobbying as the most influential, whereas conflict tactics, such as protests, were least effective (Salcido & Seck, 1992).

Colby and Buffum (1998) examined the role of NASW sponsored Political Action for Candidate Election (PACE) committees in the 1992 election. The study found the PACE committees to be very active, but questioned their overall effectiveness, especially in comparison to other political action committees. The authors recommended that PACE committees be more accountable to NASW membership and engage NASW members more directly in the support of candidates (Colby & Buffum, 1998).

Hartnett and colleagues (2005) examined the role of NASW chapters in promoting advocacy. They surveyed 22 NASW chapters and found that state chapters did attempt to make policy practice a priority, with 100% reporting that members were encouraged to engage in advocacy (Hartnett et al., 2005). Their study found that for members, time constraints limited their ability to be involved in policy practice, but that technology, such as e-mail, could enhance communication with members (Hartnett et al., 2005). Unfortunately, the study was hampered by a rather weak response rate, with only 38% of chapters returning the survey.

A further analysis by Scanlon and colleagues found that the most common political advocacy activities undertaken by NASW chapters included joining coalitions (95%), lobbying (91%), encouraging members to run for office (90%), tracking legislation (86%), and endorsing candidates (82%). Policy priorities were most commonly established through PACE committees in consultation with lobbyists or liaisons (Scanlon et al., 2006).

Lane and colleagues (2012) describe one school's involvement with preparing social work students for social action. Among the strategies the school used was a lobby/learn trip to the state capitol sponsored by NASW. Interestingly, the school seems to have developed strategies for social action independent of the state chapter of NASW (Lane et al., 2012).

A more collaborative strategy was reported by Kilbane and colleagues (2013), where a school of social work partnered with the state chapter of NASW to develop a week-long advocacy training prior to their state's legislative advocacy day. The impact on students was positive. An evaluation of the event found that students' experienced a better understanding of the relationship between policy and advocacy as well as the centrality of advocacy to the social work profession (Kilbane et al., 2013).

The present study extends the existing literature in three important ways. First, previous research did not specifically focus on the involvement of students in NASW advocacy efforts (Salcido & Seck, 1992). In addition, some studies were hampered by low response rates (Hartnett et al., 2005; Scanlon et al., 2006). Finally, previous studies have not specifically explored the question of how legislative advocacy days are used to engage social workers and students. This study will begin to fill some of those gaps.

METHOD

The study consisted of a cross-sectional survey that examined how NASW chapters engage members in policy practice. The survey was designed and implemented electronically using Survey Monkey. The sample for the study included 52 chapters of NASW (all 50 states, New York City, and Washington, DC). Permission to conduct the study was obtained through NASW and NASW assisted with the dissemination of the survey to chapter contacts. The items in the survey focused on three main topics: (1) how chapters engage social work professionals in policy practice; (2) how chapters engage social work students in policy practice; and (3) how chapters use legislative advocacy days as a tool to build policy practice skills. Data from the surveys were exported to SPSS for descriptive analysis.

RESULTS

Forty state-level chapters responded to the survey for a response rate of 76.9%. The individuals completing the survey were either NASW chapter elected leaders or paid staff. The majority of respondents reported that they were the chapter executive director (82.5%). The remaining responses were received from a chapter president (2.5%), other chapter officers (7.5%), or the chapter advocacy coordinators or directors (7.5%).

Engagement of Professionals in Advocacy

The first question that the survey sought to answer was how state chapters of NASW engage social workers in legislative advocacy. Overall, it appears that chapters involved their members in political advocacy in numerous ways (see Table 1). Almost all chapters (95.0%) reported that they e-mail members encouraging them to advocate for or against specific pieces of legislation. The majority of chapters (87.5%) reported that they form coalitions with allied organizations, support candidates through PACE committees (85.0%), develop policy positions (80.0%), and organize social workers to testify on specific pieces of legislation (80.0%). Less common strategies were efforts to organize rallies (32.5%) or use press releases directed to the media (30.0%).

One respondent volunteered that the NASW chapter reviews every piece of legislation introduced to their state legislature and they typically took a position on about 20% of the bills. The policy positions were then shared with legislators, coalition partners, NASW members, students and others. Other chapters shared that they used social media, including Facebook, Twitter, blogs, and LinkedIn, as a strategy to connect with members and keep them updated on the legislative activities of their chapter.

TABLE 1 NASW Chapter Involvement in Political Advocacy ($n = 40$)

NASW chapter involvement in political advocacy ($n = 40$)	Count	Percent
Organize and host workshops on legislative issues.	29	72.5%
Develop policy positions.	32	80.0%
Endorse and support candidates through PACE (Political Action for Candidate Election) committees.	34	85.0%
Email members to advocate for or against specific pieces of legislation.	38	95.0%
Coordinate a legislative advocacy network or committee.	35	87.5%
Organize rallies in support of or against specific pieces of legislation.	13	32.5%
Send out press releases stating the chapter's position on legislation.	12	30.0%
Coordinate social workers to testify at the state legislature.	32	80.0%
Coordinate small group meetings with legislators.	27	67.5%
Coordinate advocacy efforts with other allied coalitions or groups.	35	87.5%

Most chapters (87.5%) reported that they hosted a Legislative Action Committee to organize advocacy efforts in their state. The main activities of the Legislative Action Committees were to organize legislative advocacy days (65.7%), coordinate with other organizations and coalitions for legislative action (71.4%), and provide trainings to members on legislative advocacy (65.7%). Several chapters volunteered that their Legislative Action Committees primarily focused on promoting legislative priorities, including developing a legislative agenda, formulating positions on pending legislation, testifying at hearings, and mobilizing members when their voice is needed.

Chapters were also asked about their perception of engagement in political advocacy within their chapter (see Table 2). When asked whether their NASW chapter provides sufficient opportunities for social workers to engage in advocacy, 82.5% of respondents either strongly agreed or somewhat agreed with that statement. State chapters recognized that for the most part advocacy efforts were local, with 85.0% agreeing with the statement that most advocacy among NASW chapter members occurred at the state level. Respondents disagreed with two other statements about the political role of NASW and the political interest of social workers. Eighty percent of respondents disagreed with the statement that providing a venue for political advocacy was not really the main purpose of their NASW chapter and 60% strongly disagreed or somewhat disagreed with the statement that social workers were not that interested in political advocacy. Finally, the majority of respondents (82.5%) felt that their chapter actively fostered political advocacy among students.

Engagement of Social Work Students in Advocacy

A second area that the survey explored was how chapters engaged students in advocacy (see Table 3). The primary way that chapters involved

TABLE 2 Perceptions of Political Advocacy Among State Chapters ($n = 40$)

	Strongly Agree	Somewhat Agree	Neither Agree nor Disagree	Somewhat Disagree	Strongly Disagree
NASW chapter provides opportunities to engage in political advocacy	55.0%	27.5%	2.5%	10.0%	5.0%
Most of the political advocacy our state's social workers engage in is at the state level	40.0%	45.0%	7.5%	7.5%	0.0%
Social workers have enough ways to be politically active without the involvement of our NASW chapter	2.6%	12.8%	7.7%	28.2%	48.7%
Providing a venue for political advocacy is not really the main purpose of our NASW chapter	0.0%	17.5%	2.5%	42.5%	37.5%
The social workers in our state are not that interested in political advocacy	2.5%	17.5%	20.0%	42.5%	17.5%
Our NASW chapter actively fosters political advocacy among social work students	47.5%	35.0%	7.5%	7.5%	2.5%

TABLE 3 Student Involvement in Chapter Advocacy ($n = 40$)

Student involvement in chapter advocacy ($n = 40$)	Count	Percent
Invite students to attend trainings and workshops on advocacy.	25	62.5%
Invite students to join legislative action committee.	26	65.0%
Involve students in legislative advocacy day.	30	75.0%
Chapter does not actively encourage student involvement.	4	10.0%

students was through their state's legislative advocacy day, or day on the hill. Seventy-five percent of chapters hosted a legislative advocacy day and all of those chapters reported that students have been involved in those events. In addition, social work students have been invited to serve on Legislative Action Committees (65.0%) and attend workshops and trainings on advocacy (62.5%). Only four chapters (10%) reported that they have not actively encouraged the participation of social work students in their advocacy efforts. Three of the four chapters were in states that are very rural and have a small population base.

One respondent shared that students were involved in several different ways within their state chapter. The chapter has had six student interns that have served as an ad-hoc legislative action committee. The student interns were involved in the review of legislation, formulating policy positions, and were involved in providing legislative testimony. The same chapter reported that they utilized a network of 20 to 40 student volunteers who were actively engaged in legislative advocacy.

Legislative Advocacy Day

The final area of focus within the survey was how chapters organize legislative advocacy days and the engagement of students in legislative advocacy days (see Table 4). Thirty (75.0%) chapters reported that they have regularly hosted a legislative advocacy day. Of those who held an advocacy day, almost all (86.7%) were an annual event. All of the respondents reported that they tracked attendance at legislative advocacy days. Attendance at the event ranged from 50 to 800 participants, with a median of 217 and mean of 285. Distribution of educational materials (100%) on policy issues or advocacy strategies and talking with legislators (93.3%) were the most common activities that occurred as part of a legislative advocacy day. In most state chapters, participants attended workshops or lectures (83.3%) and participated in chapter-organized lobbying efforts (73.3%), but fewer chapters organized rallies, marches, or demonstrations as a part of their events (33.3%).

About half of the chapters (46.7%) reported that they coordinated their advocacy day with other groups. Some of the groups that state NASW chapters coordinated with included the Children's Defense Fund, National Association for Mental Illness, state coalitions against domestic violence, coalitions against poverty, health care groups, school social workers, and colleges and universities with social work programs.

TABLE 4 States That Hold a NASW-sponsored Legislative Advocacy Day ($n = 30$)

States that hold a NASW-sponsored Legislative Advocacy Day ($n = 30$)	Count	Percent
Frequency Legislative Advocacy Day is held		
Annually	26	86.7%
Biannually	3	10.0%
Less frequently	1	3.3%
Activities that are part of Legislative Advocacy Day		
Attend rallies	10	33.3%
Attend workshops or lectures	25	83.3%
Meet with state legislators about policy issues	28	93.3%
Participate in chapter-organized lobbying efforts	22	73.3%
Receive educational material on policy issues or advocacy strategies	30	100.0%
Ways students are involved		
Attend workshops or lectures	25	83.3%
Participate in chapter-organized group lobbying efforts	22	73.3%
Meet with legislators about policy issues	27	90.0%

Involvement of Students in Advocacy Day

Respondents reported that social work students were involved with legislative advocacy days in a number of different ways. In most states, students attended meetings with legislators about policy issues (90.0%), attended workshops or lectures (83.3%), and participated in chapter-organized lobbying efforts of elected officials (73.3%).

Respondents also offered other specific ways in which they involved students in legislative advocacy days. One state reported that they have regularly held a student rally in the capitol rotunda. Students typically made signs and banners and heard from elected officials. Another state shared that they annually held student-led policy poster presentations on key state-level issues. Schools of social work within that state would select a single poster to represent their school at the state capitol. Finally, one state responded that they have given out an annual advocacy award for the school with the best advocacy project, recognizing creative and effective efforts in affecting change.

Chapters were also asked about leadership roles that social work students have had as a part of their legislative advocacy day (see Table 5). The majority (63.3%) of chapters that hold a legislative advocacy day reported that students have had a leadership position in organizing their chapter's event. The most common way that students have been involved is through the recruitment of students to attend (94.7%). Other key roles included organizing the event (78.9%), planning activities to be held (73.3%), such as workshop topics or speakers, and mobilizing community members and peers involving issues or legislation (73.7%), which provided the basis for lobbying efforts. In about half of the chapters that reported using student leaders, students conducted workshops or trainings (47.4%).

Several respondents shared that students were very involved in overseeing the advocacy day event, including registering participants, distributing materials, and setting up tables. One chapter reported that each year they recruited 40 to 70 student volunteers who, under the umbrella of their state chapter, completed a social action project. These students were also sworn in as volunteers and helped facilitate the legislative advocacy day.

TABLE 5 Leadership Roles of Students ($n = 19$)

Leadership roles of students ($n = 19$)	Count	Percent
Organize Legislative Advocacy Day event	15	78.9%
Recruit participants to attend	18	94.7%
Mobilize members and peers around issues	14	73.7%
Plan activities to be held	14	73.7%
Organize group lobbying efforts	12	63.2%
Conduct workshops/ trainings	9	47.4%

TABLE 6 Barriers to Holding a Legislative Advocacy Day (*n* = 40)

Barriers to holding a Legislative Advocacy Day (n = 10)	count	percent
Too few social workers involved with the NASW chapter	6	60.0%
Too few social work students in state	1	10.0%
Lack of funding to organize Legislative Advocacy Day	9	90.0%
Rural geography makes it difficult to organize the event	10	100.0%
Lack of interest from social work community	7	70.0%
Legislature not receptive to advocacy day events	2	20.0%

Barriers to Legislative Advocacy Days

Finally, the NASW chapters that reported they did not hold a legislative advocacy day were asked about the barriers to hosting such an event (see Table 6). The most common barrier, endorsed by 100% of the chapters, was that rural geography made it difficult to organize an event, as members lived a distance from the capitol. Other common barriers were lack of funding (90.0%), lack of interest from social work community (70.0%), and too few social workers involved with the chapter (60.0%). Several chapters volunteered that it was very difficult to get professionals to attend such an event.

DISCUSSION

The goal of this study was to add to our understanding of how NASW chapters engage professional members and social work students in legislative and political advocacy. The study includes results from a survey of 40 state NASW chapters, representing 80% of the state-level chapters in the United States. While there were some states that did not respond, this study provides a fairly complete picture of the advocacy activities of state NASW chapters around the United States, and is the first study to report on the role of legislative advocacy days as a form of legislative advocacy.

Chapter Engagement in Advocacy

The first finding from this study is that state chapters do appear to be quite engaged in legislative advocacy and are using multiple strategies to involve members in advocacy efforts. All NASW chapters but one reported using at least three different strategies to engage members in legislative advocacy. The most prominent strategies used by NASW chapters were informational e-mails to members, developing policy positions on issues, forming coalitions with like-minded organizations, and coordinating social workers to testify at the state legislature. Strategies such as rallies and press releases were less commonly used.

The vast majority of NASW chapters (87.5%) reported having a legislative action committee to direct or coordinate their advocacy efforts. The legislative action committees appear to have two key organizing roles within NASW chapters. First, the committees serve as a vehicle to develop legislative priorities, policy agendas, and policy positions. Second, the committees serve a coordinating function when action is needed to mobilize members regarding specific legislation or when key legislative testimony is sought from members.

Hoefer (2001) identifies four characteristics of effective advocacy for human service groups. Groups that want to be effective in their advocacy efforts should "be knowledgeable about and proactive in the policy process; provide timely and policy related information; build a relationship with decision-makers; and build coalitions with other interest groups and policy actors" (Hoefer, 2001, p. 3). Several of the strategies that are commonly being used by 80% or more of state chapters (building coalitions, testifying before the legislature, developing policy positions) fit with these characteristics described by Hoefer. This suggests that state chapters are using effective strategies in their advocacy efforts. In contrast, fewer than one-third of NASW chapters reported that they use rallies to support or protest against legislation. Demonstrations are viewed as one of the least effective strategies for human service groups (Hoefer, 2001), so the limited use by NASW chapters of rallies as a strategy is consistent with best practice.

Legislative Advocacy Days

A second key finding from this study is that legislative advocacy days are commonly utilized as a strategy to engage social work professionals and students in policy practice. Three-fourths of state-level NASW chapters reported that they host a legislative advocacy day, most of them on an annual basis. The legislative advocacy day events typically involve dispensing educational materials to members, hosting workshops or trainings for members, and coordinating meetings with legislators. In this way, the activities that are a part of the legislative advocacy days are similar to other chapter advocacy strategies that take place throughout the year.

Social work professionals and students appear to be actively involved in the advocacy day events. Chapters in all states reported that students were engaged in similar activities as social work professionals and several chapters reported that the number of students in attendance greatly exceeded that of social work professionals. Chapters also reported that social work students regularly assumed leadership roles in organizing the event, recruiting students, and planning activities and mobilizing community members and peers.

Student Engagement

A related finding is that social work students are very engaged in NASW advocacy efforts, particularly with legislative advocacy days. The evidence of this was apparent in two ways. First, students were very involved through the legislative advocacy days. A number of respondents volunteered that their legislative advocacy day was geared toward social work students, with students representing the majority of attendees. Students also serve in a leadership capacity in two-thirds of the states that host a legislative advocacy day, helping to organize the event. Second, some state chapters also involved students in their legislative action committees, with one chapter sharing that they had six interns and between 20 and 40 student volunteers working with their legislative action committee.

Student involvement is very heartening, as the literature shows that students who build their skills in advocacy while in school have greater intention to continue to engage in advocacy after they graduate and begin their professional career (author, 2014; Butler & Coleman, 1997; Manalo, 2004; Tower & Hartnett, 2011). Participation in advocacy as a student can help to reinforce the role of advocacy within the profession (Comerford, 2003). Attending a legislative advocacy day can also build a student's sense of external political efficacy, or one's belief in the political system's responsiveness to citizen actions (Andrews, 1998). Belief that change is possible can be influential in sustaining student involvement in advocacy (Byers & Stone, 1999). If social workers perceive that their efforts will not make much of a difference, it can influence their decisions to advocate in the future (Beimers, 2014).

Barriers to Advocacy

One concern is that 25% of the states reported that they do not hold a legislative advocacy day, with geography, funding, and interest being the main barriers to holding an event. Interestingly, only one state chapter reported that too few students was a barrier to holding a legislative advocacy day event, indicating that lack of interest is found among professionals as opposed to students. There are several concerns with state NASW chapters not hosting an event. First, legislative advocacy events are a good way to introduce social work students to the social work advocacy and give them an opportunity to practice their advocacy skills. Ritter (2007, p. 355) suggests "social work students should have the opportunity to practice advocacy skills in the same way that they are given the opportunity to practice clinical skills." Schools of social work need to provide students with this opportunity and should work with NASW to overcome those barriers.

A second concern is that legislatures rely on the expertise of social work professionals in crafting social welfare policy. Legislative advocacy days help connect current and future social work professionals to their legislators. Working with legislators on policy issues is a key strategy for human service agencies to effect change (Hoefer, 2001). Introducing social work students to legislators and reconnecting professionals with their legislative representatives can initiate conversations and form relationships that can ultimately inform social policy.

Implications for Social Work Education

As a whole, these findings have important implications for social work education. Social work programs are charged with developing students into competent policy practitioners who work for social justice across client systems. Although it is not the role of NASW to train social work students, state chapters do have a vested interest in seeing social work students and professionals as active, engaged, and effective advocates. This study shows that NASW chapters are very active in engaging students and professionals in advocacy efforts. These findings suggest that schools of social work can and should continue to partner with NASW to further develop advocacy skills.

One of the key ways that NASW connects with social work students and contributes to their development as policy practitioners is through participation in legislative advocacy day events. Two approaches can be used to engage students in a legislative advocacy day, one that is university driven and one that is chapter driven.

University-driven approach. DeRigne and colleagues (2014) provide examples of how Barry University and Florida Atlantic University have built participation in their state's legislative advocacy day into the curriculum of their social work programs and have empowered student groups to provide leadership in preparing for that event. Florida Atlantic even offers an elective course where students carry out a policy practice project and are required to attend their legislative advocacy day.

Kilbane and colleagues (2013) provide a description of how Loyola University Chicago prepares clinical social work students to be effective advocates. The Illinois chapter of NASW partnered with the school of social work to develop a week-long program that included both faculty and NASW staff. The advocacy week program included workshops on the relationship of policy to practice, presentations on the legislative process, and workshops on advocacy strategies and being an effective lobbyist (Kilbane et al., 2013).

Another example is from California State University, Los Angeles, where students have an assignment to attend their NASW Legislative Lobby Day and lobby a state legislator on an NASW legislative issue or issue of their own choosing (Manalo, 2004). An evaluation of the course found that the experience had a profound influence on the likelihood of students to lobby their legislator in the future (Manalo, 2004).

Chapter-driven approach. Several respondents to the present study provided examples of chapter-driven approaches to integrating legislative advocacy days into the curriculum. One state reported that their NASW chapter hosts an annual policy poster competition. Each school in the state is invited to have one student represent their school and the students present their posters to the audience of 400–500 attendees. The chapter reported that many schools of social work have incorporated the policy poster development as a class project with the best poster being selected for presentation at their legislative advocacy day. Another state reported that they use student liaisons from each school to help organize their legislative advocacy day, recruit students, and prepare students for advocacy activities. The liaisons attend a one-day training and then serve as the point person on their campus in preparing for the legislative advocacy day.

However, chapters are also involving students in advocacy efforts throughout the year as volunteers, interns, and committee members. Chapters shared that students in some states are involved in reviewing legislation, formulating policy positions, and testifying before committees. The findings here show that in many states, NASW and schools of social work have recognized that working together as partners, there are numerous creative ways that students can be involved in advocacy efforts. Leadership within state NASW chapters and leaders of schools of social work should continue to work together to develop creative, interesting, and engaging ways of introducing social work students to policy practice. Further, states chapters should promote and share their strategies with other state chapters, building the knowledge base of policy practice.

CONCLUSION

This study reports on how chapters of NASW engage professional members and social work students in legislative and political advocacy. The findings suggest that state NASW chapters are engaged in legislative advocacy and are actively involving social work students and members in advocacy efforts. This is consistent with research, as membership in NASW has been connected to increased political participation among social workers (Hamilton & Fauri, 2001; Ritter, 2007; Ritter, 2008).

Social work has a long-standing commitment to promoting social policies that advance social and economic justice. While social work educators have a key role in preparing students to be effective advocates, professional membership is a key way to maintain that focus on advocacy beyond the walls of the classroom. NASW and schools of social work need to work hand in hand to continue strengthening the advocacy role of NASW members. Schools of social work should continue to reach out to NASW and explore creative ways to engage students in advocacy efforts and NASW should continue to work with schools of social work to ensure that our next generation of social workers are effective, engaged policy practitioners.

ACKNOWLEDGMENTS

I would like to thank Eowyn Gatlin, who as a Graduate Assistant assisted with data collection.

REFERENCES

Anderson, D. K., & Harris, B. M. (2005). Teaching social welfare policy: A comparison of two pedagogical approaches. *Journal of Social Work Education, 41*(3), 511–526.

Andrews, A. B. (1998). An exploratory study of political attitudes and acts among child and family service workers. *Children and Youth Services Review, 20*(5), 435–461.

Beimers, D. (2014). *Legislative advocacy days: Building political self-efficacy in social work students*. Manuscript submitted for publication. Minnesota State University, Mankato, MN.

Bernklau Halvor, C. D. (2012). Increasing social work students' political interest and efficacy: The experience and impact of a social welfare policy course from the students' perspective. *Dissertation Abstracts International, A: The Humanities and Social Sciences*. (Accession No. 1322719733; 201302698)

Butler, S. S., & Coleman, P. A. (1997). Raising our voices: A macro practice assignment. *Journal of Teaching in Social Work, 15*(1-2), 63–80.

Byers, K., & Stone, G. (1999). Roots of activism: A qualitative study of BSW students. *Journal of Baccalaureate Social Work, 5*(1), 1–14.

Colby, I. C., & Buffum, W. E. (1998). Social workers and PACs: An examination of National Association of Social Workers P.A.C.E. Committees. *Journal of Community Practice, 5*(4), 87–103.

Comerford, S. A. (2003). Confronting power: Undergraduates engage the legislative process in Vermont. *The Social Policy Journal, 2*(2-3), 123–143.

Council on Social Work Education. (2012). Educational Policy and Accreditation Standards. Retrieved from http://www.cswe.org/File.aspx?id=41861

DeRigne, L., Rosenwald, M., & Naranjo, F. A. (2014). Legislative advocacy and social work education: Models and new strategies. *Journal of Policy Practice, 13*(4), 316–327.

Edwards, H. R., & Hoefer, R. (2010). Are social work advocacy groups using web 2.0 effectively? *Journal of Policy Practice, 9*(3/4), 220–239.

Ezell, M. (1993). The political advocacy of social workers. *Journal of Sociology and Social Welfare, 20*(4), 81–97.

Ezell, M. (2001). *Advocacy in the human services*. Stamford, CT: Brooks/Cole.

Fitzgerald, E., & McNutt, J. (1999). Electronic advocacy in policy practice: A framework for teaching technologically based practice. *Journal of Social Work Education, 35*(3), 331–341.

Hamilton, D., & Fauri, D. (2001). Social workers' political participation: Strengthening the political confidence of social work students. *Journal of Social Work Education, 37*(2), 321-321.

Hartnett, H., Harding, S., & Scanlon, E. (2005). NASW chapters: Directors' perceptions of factors which impede and encourage active member participation. *Journal of Community Practice, 13*(4), 69-83.

Hoefer, R. (2000). Human services interest groups in four states. *Journal of Community Practice, 7*(4), 77-94.

Hoefer, R. (2001). Highly effective human services interest groups. *Journal of Community Practice, 9*(2), 1-13.

Hoefer, R. (2005). Altering state policy: Interest group effectiveness among state-level advocacy groups. *Social Work, 50*(3), 219-227.

Jackson-Elmoore, C. (2005). Informing state policymakers: Opportunities for social workers. *Social Work, 50*(3), 251-261.

Jackson-Elmoore, C. (2006). Influencing state policy: Information, access and timing. *American Journal of Health Education, 37*(3), 159-169.

Kilbane, T., Pryce, J., & Hong, P. Y. P. (2013). Advocacy week: A model to prepare clinical social workers for lobby day. *Journal of Social Work Education, 49*(1), 173-179.

Lane, S. R., Altman, J. C., Schaffner Goldberg, G., Kagotho, N., Palley, E., & Paul, M. S. (2012). Inspiring and training students for social action: Renewing a needed tradition. *Journal of Teaching in Social Work, 32*(5), 532-549.

Manalo, V. (2004). Teaching policy advocacy through state legislative and local ballot-based advocacy assignments. *The Social Policy Journal, 3*(4), 53-67.

National Association of Social Workers (NASW) (2008). *Code of Ethics.* Retrieved from https://www.socialworkers.org/pubs/code/code.asp

Powell, J. Y., & Causby, V. D. (1994). From the classroom to the capitol-from MSW students to advocates: Learning by doing. *Journal of Teaching in Social Work, 9*(1/2), 141-154.

Ritter, J. A. (2007). Evaluating the political participation of licensed social workers in the new millennium. *Journal of Policy Practice, 6*(4), 61-78.

Ritter, J. A. (2008). A national study predicting licensed social workers' levels of political participation: The role of resources, psychological engagement, and recruitment networks. *Social Work, 53*(4), 347-357.

Rocha, C. J. (2000). Evaluating experiential teaching methods in a policy practice course: The case for service learning to increase political participation. *Journal of Social Work Education, 36*(1), 53-63.

Rocha, C., Poe, B., & Thomas, V. (2010). Political activities of social workers: Addressing perceived barriers to political participation. *Social Work, 55,* 317-325.

Rome, S. H., & Hoechstetter, S. (2010). Social work and civic engagement: The political participation of professional social workers. *Journal of Sociology & Social Welfare, 37,* 107.

Salcido, R. M., & Seck, E. T. (1992). Political participation among social work chapters. *Social Work, 37*(6), 563-564.

Saulnier, C. F. (2000). Policy practice. *Journal of Teaching in Social Work, 20*(1-2), 121-144. doi:10.1300/J067v20n01_08

Scanlon, E., Hartnett, H., & Harding, S. (2006). An analysis of the political activities of NASW state chapters. *Journal of Policy Practice*, *5*(4), 41–54.

Teater, B. (2008). "Your agenda is our agenda": State legislators' perspectives of interest group influence on political decision making. *Journal of Community Practice*, *16*(2), 201–220.

Tower, L. E., & Hartnett, H. P. (2011). An Internet-based assignment to teach students to engage in policy practice: A three-cohort study. *Journal of Policy Practice*, *10*(1), 65–77.

Tower, L. E., & Hash, K. M. (2013). "Hearing the real stories about the issues at hand": Politically active elders engage bachelor in social work (BSW) students in influencing social policy. *Social Work Education*, *32*(7), 920–932.

Weaver, R. D., & Nackerud, L. G. (2005). Evaluating the effects of an applied learning exercise on students' interest in social policy. *Journal of Teaching in Social Work*, *25*(3), 105–120.

Weiss, I., Gal, J., & Katan, J. (2006). Social policy for social work: A teaching agenda. *British Journal of Social Work*, *36*(5), 789–806.

Wolk, J. L. (1981). Are social workers politically active? *Social Work*, *26*(4), 283–288.

Human Rights and the Social Work Curriculum: Integrating Human Rights into Skill-Based Education Regarding Policy Practice Behaviors

JULIE A. STEEN and MARY MANN
School of Social Work, University of Central Florida, Orlando, Florida, USA

This article provides a model for social work educators seeking to integrate human rights content in the policy course. Each of the four policy-related practice behaviors (e.g., policy formulation, policy analysis, policy advocacy, and collaboration in policy practice) is examined with respect to the traditional methods used in social welfare policy courses and the ways in which these methods can be expanded to include human rights content. Available literature and multimedia resources are noted and practical human rights applications are presented with the goal of supporting efforts to achieve this integration.

During the past two decades, leaders within the social work profession have begun to integrate human rights content into social work literature, positions of professional associations, and educational accreditation standards. The connection between social work and human rights has been firmly established in the literature (Healy, 2008a; Ife, 2001; Reichert, 2003, 2006; Steen, 2006; Witkin, 1998; Wronka, 2008). Professional associations, such as the International Federation of Social Workers (2012a; 2012b), have integrated human rights concepts into professional definitions and ethical principles. Spurred by these advancements, social work educators have begun to integrate the human rights philosophy into the social work curriculum. This entry into the educational sphere can be seen in the work of both international and national entities representing social work education, namely the

International Association of Schools of Social Work (2004) and its American counterpart, the Council on Social Work Education (2008).

Of most importance to this discussion is the way in which the Council on Social Work Education (CSWE) has integrated human rights concepts into accreditation standards. In the most recent version of the Educational Policy and Accreditation Standards (EPAS), CSWE (2008) established 10 competencies for social work education. Included in these standards are two competencies relevant to this manuscript. The first is the human rights competency (Educational Policy 2.1.5), which reads as follows:

> **Advance human rights and social and economic justice.** Each person, regardless of position in society, has basic human rights, such as freedom, safety, privacy, an adequate standard of living, health care, and education. Social workers recognize the global interconnections of oppression and are knowledgeable about theories of justice and strategies to promote human and civil rights. Social work incorporates social justice practice in organizations, institutions, and society to ensure that these basic human rights are distributed equitably and without prejudice. (CSWE, 2008, p. 5)

This human rights content is a natural fit for the policy sequence, which is guided by the following policy competency (Educational Policy 2.1.8):

> **Engage in policy practice to advance social and economic wellbeing and to deliver effective social work services.** Social work practitioners understand that policy affects service delivery, and they actively engage in policy practice. Social workers know the history and current structures of social policies and services; the role of policy in service delivery; and the role of practice in policy development. (CSWE, 2008, p. 6)

In light of the natural fit between these two competencies, an examination of methods for integrating the two content areas is warranted.

This relationship between the two competencies is examined best at the ground level where the concepts are applied in practice. Thus, this manuscript goes beyond the conceptual level and focuses on practice behaviors, which are operationalizations of the competency in the practice world. The policy competency (Educational Policy 2.1.8) is operationalized into four basic skill-based elements: policy formulation, policy analysis, policy advocacy, and "collaboration with colleagues and clients" (CSWE, 2008, p. 6) during the policy process. In this manuscript, we provide social work educators with a guide for presenting and applying human rights content in educational efforts focused on these four policy practice behaviors.

POLICY FORMULATION

The policy formulation process is one of the traditional subjects addressed in policy courses (Barusch, 2014; Cummins, Byers, & Pedrick, 2011; DiNitto, 2011; Haynes & Mickelson, 2009; Jansson, 2013; Karger & Stoesz, 2013; Segal, 2013). However, social work texts in the policy field focus almost exclusively on American policy-making bodies. A few authors do include a chapter regarding international policy, but this material is often presented in a compartmentalized fashion. The separation of domestic and international policy content may be one inhibitor to the full integration of human rights concepts in the policy course. Actors in the international level of policy development are well versed in the human rights philosophy and actively use human rights terms in the construction of policy. Further, policy debates at the international level and the international policies themselves have an influence on domestic policies. A more thorough integration of international policy development in the policy course is one way to broaden student awareness of the human rights philosophy, while deepening their understanding of policy development in an increasingly global context.

Human rights content can be integrated into policy courses through the use of examples of human rights policies that develop at the international level and influence policy development at the domestic level. One of the primary ways that human rights content becomes embedded in American policy is through the interactions between the United Nations and the U.S. Congress. When the United Nations adopts a human rights convention, the convention then moves to the national policy-making institutions of the member nations. At this point, the national policy-making institution can ratify or reject the convention. Nations may be required or encouraged to establish national policy that brings them in compliance with the convention. Examinations of this process should also include a consideration of the ways in which national policy may influence international human rights policy. The following section provides an example of this interaction in the development of human rights policy.

Policy Formulation—Human Rights Application

The influence of international human rights policy on national human rights policy can be demonstrated through the formulation of human trafficking law. U.S. policies regarding human trafficking, namely the Victims of Trafficking and Violence Prevention Act of 2000 and its subsequent amendments, are often examined in a narrow domestic context (Bromfield & Capous-Desyllas, 2012). Though domestic institutions and interest groups had significant impacts on the form that this policy took, the origin of this policy is strongly rooted in the work of international institutions.

In the late 1990s, the United Nations turned its attention to the problem of human trafficking and addressed this issue through the adoption of the Convention against Transnational Organized Crime and an accompanying protocol titled Protocol to Prevent, Suppress and Punish Trafficking in Persons, especially Women and Children. This effort was initiated following a request by Argentina at the 1997 Session of the United Nations Commission on Crime Prevention and Criminal Justice (Gallagher, 2001). The resulting Protocol, adopted in 2000 by the United Nations, established the following conditions for member nations that ratify the Protocol:

- adoption of laws that criminalize trafficking;
- provision of services to victims of trafficking;
- expansion of victims' opportunities to remain in the country;
- facilitation of victims' safe return to country of origin;
- prevention of trafficking activity;
- improvement of law enforcement response through training and cross-departmental communication;
- integration of border control and trafficking prevention efforts; and
- prevention of fraud in the area of identification and travel documentation. (United Nations Office on Drugs and Crime, 2004)

The U.S. policy, Victims of Trafficking and Violence Prevention Act of 2000, closely mirrored the United Nations Protocol. The Act established a national task force to facilitate a cross-departmental response to the problem, mandated the provision of prevention programs in both international and domestic venues, expanded victims' access to benefits and services, expanded victims' opportunities to remain in the United States, expanded training for law enforcement, expanded definitions of trafficking in criminal statutes, and increased sentencing for these crimes. In addition to these provisions, the U.S. policy established a process by which nations were evaluated with regard to their commitment to prevent and address human trafficking. If a nation failed to demonstrate a sufficient response to the problem, the policy allowed U.S. officials to sever aid to the country (U.S. Department of State, n.d.).

The relationship between the policy development processes of national and international institutions is evident in the formation of this human rights policy. The United Nations began work on the Protocol following the 1997 request by Argentina. In 1998, President Clinton issued a call to action in his Memorandum on Steps to Combat Violence Against Women and Trafficking in Women and Girls. The U.S. Congress began holding hearings regarding the issue in 1999 (Stolz, 2007). While the U.S. policy was passing through the legislative process, the Clinton Administration was engaged in negotiations with the United Nations regarding the details of the Protocol (Defeis, 2004). These simultaneous processes should not be viewed as separate and distinct policy formulations, but as interactions between national and international institutions (Stolz, 2005). Thus, this human rights policy provides students with the opportunity to examine policy formulation in a multi-level, institutional context.

POLICY ANALYSIS

Policy analysis is the second major area of emphasis in the policy-related practice behaviors advanced by CSWE (2008). Since the science of policy analysis has a rich foundation with a variety of methods, the social work literature includes several different approaches to teaching this skill. Some of these approaches are technical in nature. Examples include impact analysis and cost-benefit analysis (Caputo, 2014; O'Connor & Netting, 2010). This type of technical skill building is paramount for expanding students' capacity for critical thought and attention to detail. However, another important aspect of policy analysis is the moral assessment of the actions required by the policy and the impacts created by the policy's mandates. This second approach to policy analysis relies on a set of standards, typically derived from moral philosophies or professional codes (Jansson, 2012). It is this second approach where human rights content can be most easily integrated into skill-based education regarding policy analysis.

Concepts from international human rights agreements can serve as key standards by which policies are analyzed (Hokenstad, Healy, Libal, & Law, 2012; Reichert, 2003; van Wormer, 2004). These core human rights concepts can be found in a variety of forms, such as resolutions, which have been adopted by the United Nations General Assembly, and conventions, which have been signed and ratified by a number of member nations. While there is considerable difference in the implementation process for resolutions and conventions, they both provide standards by which local, state, and national policies may be analyzed. Further, these standards are provided for many areas of social welfare policy, such as child welfare, juvenile justice, and mental health. See Table 1 for a list of select human rights agreements that can serve as frameworks for policy analysis. The next section provides an example of a policy analysis based on standards from human rights agreements.

Policy Analysis—Human Rights Application

The integration of human rights content in policy analysis can be demonstrated through the evaluation of health care policy. Human rights standards for the field of health care are established in the International Covenant on Economic, Social and Cultural Rights (United Nations, 1966). Article 12 of this Covenant reads as follows: "the States Parties to the present Covenant recognize the right of everyone to the enjoyment of the highest attainable standard

TABLE 1 Select List of International Human Rights Documents

Subject	Title of Human Rights Document
Aging	*Principles for Older Persons*
Child Welfare	*Convention on the Rights of the Child*
Disability	*Convention on the Rights of Persons with Disabilities; Declaration on the Rights of Mentally Retarded Persons; Declaration on the Rights of Disabled Persons; Standard Rules on the Equalization of Opportunities for Persons with Disabilities*
GLBT	*Statement on Human Rights, Sexual Orientation and Gender Identity*
Juvenile Justice	*Standard Minimum Rules for the Administration of Juvenile Justice (Beijing Rules); Guidelines for the Prevention of Juvenile Delinquency (Riyadh Guidelines)*
Labor	*Employment Policy Convention; International Convention on the Protection of the Rights of All Migrant Workers and Members of their Families; Worst Forms of Child Labour Convention; Protocol to Prevent, Suppress and Punish Trafficking in Persons Especially Women and Children*
Mental Health	*Principles for the Protection of Persons with Mental Illness and the Improvement of Mental Health*
Poverty	*Universal Declaration on the Eradication of Hunger and Malnutrition;*
Race and Ethnicity	*International Convention on the Elimination of All Forms of Racial Discrimination; Indigenous and Tribal Peoples Convention; Durban Declaration and Programme of Action; Declaration on the Rights of Indigenous Peoples; Declaration on the Rights of Persons Belonging to National or Ethnic, Religions, and Linguistic Minorities*
Refugees	*Convention relating to the Status of Refugees; Declaration on the Human Rights of Individuals Who are not Nationals of the Country in which They Live*
Women	*Convention on the Elimination of All Forms of Discrimination against Women; Declaration on the Elimination of Violence against Women*

of physical and mental health" (United Nations, 1966, Article 12.1). The dimensions of this human right are further outlined in a publication of the United Nations Economic and Social Council (2000) titled *Substantive Issues Arising in the Implementation of the International Covenant on Economic, Social and Cultural Rights*. Based on this publication, health care policy should ensure availability, accessibility, acceptability, and quality. The concept of availability represents the presence of health services and the concept of accessibility represents the degree to which these services are open to all. Acceptability refers to alignment with ethical standards, whereas quality refers to alignment with technical standards.

These four dimensions of the human right to health provide a framework for an analysis of American health care policy. An example of this type of analysis can be found in the work of Gable (2011), who analyzed the Patient Protection and Affordable Care Act in terms of the human right to health. The Act supports accessibility through several provisions, such as the expansion of Medicaid and the expansion of private insurance coverage for pre-existing conditions. This increase in access can directly affect health, as evidenced by research that links Medicaid expansion to reduced mortality (Sommers, Baicker, & Epstein, 2012). Though the primary goal of the Act was to increase access, analysts have also assessed the Act using the remaining three standards of availability, acceptability, and quality. Both Furrow (2011) and Gable (2011) argue that the Act's quality improvement provisions increase the system's attention to technical/scientific standards of care. Gable also cites provisions that may ensure availability by increasing supports for those entering health professions. Further, acceptability is enhanced through the Act's promotion of culturally competent practice (Teitelbaum, Cartwright-Smith, & Rosenbaum, 2012). Though the system created by this Act will not achieve perfect alignment with all four of the human rights standards, the provisions do support improvement in each of these four areas.

POLICY ADVOCACY

Policy advocacy is another component of CSWE's (2008) policy-related practice behaviors. Social work has a long history of engagement in both case advocacy and cause advocacy, though the majority of educational materials and activities focus on cause advocacy. Cause advocacy, which involves the advancement of a particular policy, is primarily taught with an emphasis on legislative advocacy (Cummins et al., 2011; Haynes & Mickelson, 2009; Jansson, 2013). This facet of social work education is supported by a strong infrastructure of legislative materials from Influencing State Policy (n.d.), a network of social work educators who teach social welfare policy. Educators who teach this material often incorporate state-level Lobby Day activities into their courses (Manalo, 2004; Powell & Causby, 1994). Case advocacy, which involves the advancement of a just application of policy to an individual case, receives less emphasis in social work education, but materials are available to support this method (Hoefer, 2011; Lens, 2004; Schneider & Lester, 2001). In sum, social work educators have access to a wide array of resources for teaching advocacy skills.

These resources extend into the human rights arena. Social work authors have integrated human rights applications in their advocacy-related publications to an extent that is far greater than for any other practice behavior. The social work literature includes guides for advocacy within the United Nations (Healy, 2008b; Healy & Link, 2011; Pollack, 2007). Similar to the state-level Lobby Day events, the United Nations hosts a Social Work Day every spring (Nadkarni, 2013). Social work students from a wide variety of universities travel to New York to attend this event, meet international human rights leaders, and strengthen their understanding of the United Nations' structure and process. These resources provide a strong foundation for instruction regarding cause-based advocacy.

While most of the literature focuses on cause-based advocacy, several opportunities exist on the international level for case-based advocacy. Individual complaints regarding human rights violations can be submitted to international entities for review. Some of these entities are connected to human rights conventions, such as the International Covenant on Civil and Political Rights; the Convention against Torture and Other Cruel, Inhuman or Degrading Treatment or Punishment; the Convention on the Elimination of All Forms of Racial Discrimination; and the Convention on the Elimination of All Forms of Discrimination Against Women. These conventions are connected to a monitoring entity, which is responsible for receiving and reviewing individual complaints (Bayefsky, 2003). In addition to these entities, there are regional human rights commissions, such as the European Commission of Human Rights (van Dijk & van Hoof, 1998) and the Inter-American Commission on Human Rights (Davidson, 1997; Medina, 1990). A case heard before the Inter-American Commission on Human Rights is featured in an article by Gammonley, Rotabi, Forte, and Martin (2013), who provide a model for integrating both case-based and cause-based human rights advocacy in social work education.

Policy Advocacy—Human Rights Application

The integration of human rights content can be demonstrated in both case-based and cause-based advocacy. This application will focus on case-based advocacy. Please see the fourth section regarding collaboration for an application of human rights content in cause-based advocacy.

Case-based human rights advocacy can be demonstrated through the work of Mental Disability Rights International and the Center for Justice and International Law on behalf of Jorge Bernal and Julio César Rotela. Both of these young men spent years living in the Neuro-Psychiatric Hospital of Paraguay, an institution housing individuals with autism and similar disorders (Hillman, 2005). They had been "kept for more than four years in solitary confinement in small cells, naked, and without access to the bathrooms" (Inter-American Commission on Human Rights, 2003, para. 60). "The cells reeked of urine and feces, and the cell walls were smeared with excrement. Each boy spent approximately four hours of every other day in an outdoor pen, which was littered with human excrement, garbage, and broken glass" (Disability Rights International, 2014, para. 4). Mental Disability Rights International filmed these conditions and joined with Witness to bring these violations to the public's attention (Witness, n.d.).

Mental Disability Rights International and the Center for Justice and International Law brought the case before the Inter-American Commission on Human Rights, which ruled in favor of the two young men and called for Paraguay to immediately respond to the situation (Disability Rights International, 2014; Inter-American Commission on Human Rights, 2003). This advocacy resulted in improved community-based care for Mr. Bernal, slightly improved institutional care for Mr. Rotela, and a broader effort to improve mental health systems within Paraguay (Disability Rights International, 2014). A video that summarizes this advocacy effort is publicly available on vimeo (Disability Rights International, 2011).

COLLABORATION

The last component of the policy-related practice behaviors involves "collaboration with colleagues and clients" (CSWE, 2008, p. 6) during the policy process. This topic is relatively new to the policy sequence and has just recently been integrated into several policy texts. Chapin's (2011) text provides the most comprehensive treatment of this subject. She guides students in the performance of two key collaborative tasks: eliciting client perceptions and preferences in the analysis and formulation of policy and joining with colleagues in advocacy efforts.

Human rights content is relevant to the practice of collaboration and ultimately strengthens this practice. This connection between human rights and collaboration is expressed in two ways. First, policy practitioners can include human rights advocacy agencies as partners in collaborative efforts designed to change policy. Unfortunately, these non-governmental organizations are often misunderstood, as some believe that they focus only on human rights violations stemming from war and political violence. The reality is that many of these human rights agencies embrace the full range of human rights. Notable examples include Amnesty International's campaigns to protect Native American women from sexual violence and reduce maternal and infant mortality in the United States (Amnesty International, 2007; 2010). Other important advocacy organizations include Child Rights International Network, Human Rights Watch, and the International Committee of the Red Cross. The second way in which human rights relates to collaboration involves the charge to include clients in the process. Within the international human rights community, this participation has been conceptualized as a human right (Bessell & Gal, 2009; Secker, 2009). Human rights documents explicitly promote the right to participate in decision making at both societal and personal levels. This right is advanced for a wide variety of populations, including children, people with disabilities, and elders. A list of several human rights documents and their statements regarding this right can be found in Table 2.

TABLE 2 Statements Regarding the Human Right to Participation

Subject	Title of Human Rights Document	Statements regarding Participation Rights
Aging	*Principles for Older Persons*	"Older persons should be able to participate in determining when and at what pace withdrawal from the labour force takes place."
		"Older persons should remain integrated in society, participate actively in the formulation and implementation of policies that directly affect their well-being and share their knowledge and skills with younger generations."
		"Older persons should be able to form movements or associations of older persons."
		"Older persons should be able to enjoy human rights and fundamental freedoms when residing in any shelter, care or treatment facility, including full respect for their dignity, beliefs, needs and privacy and for the right to make decisions about their care and the quality of their lives."
Child Welfare	*Convention on the Rights of the Child*	"States Parties shall assure to the child who is capable of forming his or her own views the right to express those views freely in all matters affecting the child, the views of the child being given due weight in accordance with the age and maturity of the child."
		"For this purpose, the child shall in particular be provided the opportunity to be heard in any judicial and administrative proceedings affecting the child, either directly, or through a representative or an appropriate body, in a manner consistent with the procedural rules of national law."
		"States Parties recognize the rights of the child to freedom of association and to freedom of peaceful assembly."
Disability	*Standard Rules on the Equalization of Opportunities for Persons with Disabilities*	"Personal assistance programmes should be designed in such a way that the persons with disabilities using the programmes have a decisive influence on the way in which the programmes are delivered."
Labor	*International Convention on the Protection of the Rights of All Migrant Workers and Members of their Families*	"States Parties recognize the right of migrant workers and members of their families: to take part in meetings and activities of trade unions and of any other associations established in accordance with law."

		"Migrant workers and members of their families shall have the right to participate in public affairs of their State of origin and to vote and to be elected at elections of that State, in accordance with its legislation."
"States Parties shall consider the establishment of procedures or institutions through which account may be taken, both in States of origin and in States of employment, of special needs, aspirations and obligations of migrant workers and members of their families and shall envisage, as appropriate, the possibility for migrant workers and members of their families to have their freely chosen representatives in those institutions."
Indigenous Peoples	Indigenous and Tribal Peoples Convention	"Governments shall have the responsibility for developing, with the participation of the peoples concerned, co-ordinated and systematic action to protect the rights of these peoples and to guarantee respect for their integrity."
"The peoples concerned shall have the right to decide their own priorities for the process of development as it affects their lives, beliefs, institutions and spiritual well-being and the lands they occupy or otherwise use, and to exercise control, to the extent possible, over their own economic, social and cultural development. In addition, they shall participate in the formulation, implementation and evaluation of plans and programmes for national and regional development which may affect them directly."
"The rights of the peoples concerned to the natural resources pertaining to their lands shall be specially safeguarded. These rights include the right of these peoples to participate in the use, management and conservation of these resources."
"Procedures established by the peoples concerned for the transmission of land rights among members of these peoples shall be respected."
"The peoples concerned shall be consulted whenever consideration is being given to their capacity to alienate their lands or otherwise transmit their rights outside their own community."

Collaboration—Human Rights Application

A model for collaborative advocacy efforts can be found in the International Campaign to Ban Landmines and the Cluster Munition Coalition. In the 1990s, several international human rights advocacy organizations, including Handicap International and Human Rights Watch, joined together in an effort to ban anti-personnel mines. The coalition was involved in the full span of policy development activities: "[composing] its own draft treaty which it submitted as a model, [attending] all preparatory meetings, and [commenting] on every draft written by the Austrian delegation throughout the Ottawa Process" (Cameron, 1999, p. 92). The movement attained great success in 1997 with the adoption of the Anti-Personnel Mine Ban Convention, also known as the Ottawa Treaty. Some authors have attributed this success to the collaborative nature of the advocacy efforts, which included nation states, non-governmental human rights organizations, and citizens (Cameron, 1999; Peters, 1999). In the next decade, many of these advocates joined again in a successful campaign for the adoption of another convention focused on a similar weapon. This campaign successfully ended with the 2008 adoption of the Convention on Cluster Munitions (Borrie, 2009; Brabant, 2010; Docherty, 2012).

Survivors of war played a forceful role in advocacy for the 1997 Anti-Personnel Mine Ban Convention and the 2008 Convention on Cluster Munitions. Survivors provided testimony at key points during the advocacy process (Borrie, 2009; Brabant, 2010; Docherty, 2012). One survivor in discussing membership in this coalition stated:

> [M]embership is painful, because to be a member you must suffer true loss ... membership also brings strength, because in order to be member [sic] you agree that it is important to go beyond your pain and to strive to make a difference by using your voice and your experience to demand that countries stop using their inhumane weapons. (Handicap International, 2013, p. 22)

Their testimony had a substantial impact, as evidenced by one nation's representative who previously had opposed the ban and later wrote a letter of appreciation to the survivors who testified. In the letter, the representative writes:

> I was unaware of the terrible post conflict effects of cluster munitions .... I hope that the draft convention that we will adopt today and the contribution I have been able to make to achieving this historic goal to ban these arms that cause unacceptable harm will serve to redress the balance; so that in future [sic] civilians will not have to suffer the losses and injuries that you and your families have had to endure. (Brabant, 2010, p. 5)

This participation by survivors provides social work educators with a successful model of meaningful and empowering participation. The advocacy efforts of these survivors are featured in a video that is publicly available to educators and students through vimeo (Handicap International, 2010). Nash (2012), a coordinator of the Cluster Munition Coalition, emphasized the important components of the effort to facilitate participation, which include a "support network, peer-peer support structure or buddy system" (p. 130). A portion of this support was provided by Handicap International (2013), a human rights organization that served as a founding member of both the International Campaign to Ban Landmines and the Custer Munition Coalition. Handicap International published an extensive guide for organizations seeking to support survivors when they are engaged in advocacy efforts. The video and the guide, both available online, can serve as important resources for social work educators seeking to assist students in mastering the EPAS practice behavior regarding collaboration.

CONCLUSION

In this manuscript we illustrate how a human rights framework can enrich policy courses while meeting CSWE requirements to incorporate specific practice behaviors. The human rights framework can also assist educators in creating opportunities for students to identify and address the oftentimes myriad and intersecting issues that can contribute to human rights violations. Through the incorporation of four practice behaviors including policy formulation, policy analysis, policy advocacy, and collaboration, students can learn to simultaneously pinpoint the issues while also working to select and utilize components of these practice behaviors to respond.

Grounded in the human rights philosophy, educators can introduce existing human rights tools and instruments as guides for new policy formulation, standards for analysis of policies, or platforms for advocacy and collaboration when discussing specific human rights issues. Incorporating existing human rights tools and instruments offers opportunities to recognize and address the connections between local, national, and international concerns and highlights the increasing connectivity and impact between and among countries. In this way, the infusion of human rights furthers students' understanding of not only human rights and policy practice, but also the global level of social problems, resources, and action.

REFERENCES

Amnesty International. (2007). *Maze of injustice: The failure to protect Indigenous women from sexual violence in the USA*. New York, NY: Author. Retrieved from http://www.amnestyusa.org/pdfs/mazeofinjustice.pdf

Amnesty International. (2010). *Deadly delivery: The maternal health care crisis in the USA*. London, England: Author. Retrieved from http://www.amnestyusa.org/sites/default/files/pdfs/deadlydelivery.pdf

Barusch, A. S. (2014). *Foundations of social policy: Social justice in human perspective* (5th ed.). Belmont, CA: Brooks/Cole.

Bayefsky, A. F. (2003). *How to complain to the UN human rights treaty system*. Norwell, MA: Kluwer Law International.

Bessell, S., & Gal, T. (2009). Forming partnerships: The human rights of children in need of care and protection. *International Journal of Children's Rights, 17*, 283–298.

Borrie, J. (2009). *Unacceptable harm: A history of how the Treaty to Ban Cluster Munitions was won*. New York and Geneva: United Nations. Retrieved from http://unidir.ch/files/publications/pdfs/unacceptable-harm-a-history-of-how-the-treaty-to-ban-cluster-munitions-was-won-en-258.pdf

Brabant, S. (2010). The ban advocates: Cluster munition victims' commitment to the implementation of the Convention on Cluster Munitions. *Disarmament Forum, 1*, 1–12. Retrieved from http://www.einiras.org/Services/Digital-Library/Publications/Detail/?lng=en&id=114363

Bromfield, N. F., & Capous-Desyllas, M. (2012). Underlying motives, moral agendas and unlikely partnerships: The formulation of the U.S. Trafficking in Victims Protection Act through the data and voices of key policy players. *Advances in Social Work, 13*, 243–261.

Cameron, M. A. (1999). Global civil society and the Ottawa process: Lessons from the movement to ban anti-personnel mines. *Canadian Foreign Policy Journal, 7*, 85–102.

Caputo, R. K. (2014). *Policy analysis for social workers*. Thousand Oaks, CA: Sage.

Chapin, R. K. (2011). *Social policy for effective practice: A strengths approach* (2nd ed.). New York, NY: Routledge.

Clinton, President William J. (1998). *Memorandum on Steps to Combat Violence Against Women and Trafficking in Women and Girls*. Retrieved from http://www.gpo.gov/fdsys/pkg/WCPD-1998-03-16/pdf/WCPD-1998-03-16-Pg412.pdf

Council on Social Work Education. (2008). *Educational policy and accreditation standards*. Retrieved from http://www.cswe.org/File.aspx?id=13780

Cummins, L. K., Byers, K. V., & Pedrick, L. (2011). *Policy practice for social workers: New strategies for a new era*. Boston, MA: Allyn & Bacon.

Davidson, J. S. (1997). *The inter-American human rights system*. Brookfield, VT: Dartmouth.

Defeis, E. F. (2004). Protocol to Prevent, Suppress and Punish Trafficking in Persons—A new approach. *ILSA Journal of International & Comparative Law, 10*, 485–491.

DiNitto, D. M. (2011). *Social welfare: Politics and public policy* (7th ed.). Boston, MA: Pearson.

Disability Rights International. (2011). *United Nations documentary on DRI Paraguay advocacy*. Retrieved from http://vimeo.com/26781518

Disability Rights International. (2014). *Disability Rights International's work in Paraguay*. Retrieved from http://www.disabilityrightsintl.org/work/country-projects/paraguay/

Docherty, B. (2012). The convention on cluster munitions. In R. E. Williams & P. R. Viotti (Eds.), *Arms control: History, theory, and policy* (Vol. 1) (pp. 265–283). Santa Barbara, CA: ABC-CLIO.

Furrow, B. R. (2011). Regulating patient safety: The Patient Protection and Affordable Care Act. *University of Pennsylvania Law Review, 159*, 1727–1775.

Gable, L. (2011). The Patient Protection and Affordable Care Act, public health, and the elusive target of human rights. *Journal of Law, Medicine & Ethics, 39*, 340–354.

Gallagher, A. (2001). Human rights and the new UN protocols on trafficking and migrant smuggling: A preliminary analysis. *Human Rights Quarterly, 23*, 975–1004.

Gammonley, D., Rotabi, K. S., Forte, J., & Martin, A. (2013). Beyond study abroad: A human rights delegation to teach policy advocacy. *Journal of Social Work Education, 49*, 619–634.

Handicap International. (2010). *Ban advocates: From victims to champions* [Motion picture]. Retrieved from http://vimeo.com/8998329

Handicap International. (2013). *Advocacy with victims: Good practice and lessons learned in influencing policy*. Retrieved from http://reliefweb.int/sites/reliefweb.int/files/resources/Handicap%20international%20-Advocacy%20with%20victims.pdf

Haynes, K. S., & Mickelson, J. S. (2009). *Affecting change: Social workers in the political arena* (7th ed.). Upper Saddle River, NJ: Pearson.

Healy, L. M. (2008a). Exploring the history of social work as a human rights profession. *International Social Work, 51*, 735–748.

Healy, L. M. (2008b). *International social work: Professional action in an interdependent world* (2nd ed.). New York, NY: Oxford.

Healy, L. M., & Link, R. J. (2011). *Handbook of international social work: Human rights, development, and the global profession*. New York, NY: Oxford.

Hillman, A. A. (2005). Protecting mental disability rights: A success story in the Inter-American Human Rights System. *Human Rights Brief, 12*(3), 25–28.

Hoefer, R. (2011). *Advocacy practice for social work* (2nd ed.). Chicago, IL: Lyceum.

Hokenstad, M. C. T., Healy, L., Libal, K., & Law, C. K. (2012, July). *Teaching human rights in social work education: Global concepts and local applications*. Paper presented at the Joint World Conference on Social Work and Social Development, Stockholm, Sweden.

Ife, J. (2001). *Human rights and social work: Toward rights-based practice*. New York, NY: Cambridge University.

Influencing State Policy. (n.d.). *About us*. Retrieved from http://www.statepolicy.org/About%20Us/about%20us.html

Inter-American Commission on Human Rights. (2003). *Precautionary measures 2003*. Retrieved from http://www.cidh.org/medidas/2003.eng.htm

International Association of Schools of Social Work. (2004). *Global standards for the education and training of the social work profession*. Retrieved from http://cdn.ifsw.org/assets/ifsw_65044-3.pdf

International Federation of Social Workers. (2012a). *Definition of social work*. Retrieved from http://ifsw.org/policies/definition-of-social-work/

International Federation of Social Workers. (2012b). *Statement of ethical principles*. Retrieved from http://ifsw.org/policies/statement-of-ethical-principles/

Jansson, B. S. (2012). *The reluctant welfare state: Engaging history to advance social work practice in contemporary society* (7th ed.). Belmont, CA: Brooks/Cole.

Jansson, B. S. (2013). *Becoming an effective policy advocate: From policy practice to social justice* (7th ed.). Belmont, CA: Brooks/Cole.

Karger, H. J., & Stoesz, D. (2013). *American social welfare policy: A pluralist approach* (7th ed.). Boston, MA: Pearson.

Lens, V. (2004). Principled negotiation: A new tool for case advocacy. *Social Work, 49*, 506–513.

Manalo, V. (2004). Teaching policy advocacy through state legislative and local ballot-based advocacy assignments. *The Social Policy Journal, 3*(4), 53–67.

Medina, C. (1990). The Inter-American Commission on Human Rights and the Inter-American Court of Human Rights: Reflections on a joint venture. *Human Rights Quarterly, 12*, 439–464.

Nadkarni, V. V. (2013). IASSW and Social Work Day at the United Nations: A proud achievement. *International Social Work, 56*, 252–256.

Nash, T. (2012). Civil society and cluster munitions: Building blocks of a global campaign. In M. Kaldor, H. L. Moore, & S. Selchow (Eds.), *Global civil society 2012: Ten years of critical reflection* (pp. 124–141). Basingstoke, Hampshire, UK: Palgrave Macmillan.

O'Connor, M. K., & Netting, F. E. (2010). *Analyzing social policy: Multiple perspectives for critically understanding and evaluating policy*. Hoboken, NJ: Wiley.

Peters, A. (1999). *International partnerships on the road to ban anti-personnel landmines*. Washington, DC: Open Society Institute.

Pollack, D. (2007). Social workers and the United Nations: Effective advocacy strategies. *International Social Work, 50*, 113–119.

Powell, J. Y., & Causby, V. D. (1994). From the classroom to the capitol—From MSW students to advocates: Learning by doing. *Journal of Teaching in Social Work, 9*(1-2), 141–154.

Reichert, E. (2003). *Social work and human rights: A foundation for policy and practice*. New York, NY: Columbia University.

Reichert, E. (2006). *Understanding human rights: An exercise book*. Thousand Oaks, CA: Sage.

Secker, E. (2009). Expanding the concept of participatory rights. *The International Journal of Human Rights, 13*, 697–715.

Schneider, R. L., & Lester, L. (2001). *Social work advocacy: A new framework for action*. Stamford, CT: Brooks/Cole.

Segal, E. A. (2013). *Social welfare policy and social programs: A values perspective* (3rd ed.). Belmont, CA: Brooks/Cole.

Sommers, B. D., Baicker, K., & Epstein, A. M. (2012). Mortality and access to care among adults after state Medicaid expansions. *The New England Journal of Medicine, 367*, 1025–1034.

Steen, J. A. (2006). The roots of human rights advocacy and a call to action. *Social Work, 51*, 101–105.

Stolz, B. A. (2005). Educating policymakers and setting the criminal justice policy-making agenda: Interest groups and the "Victims of Trafficking and Violence Act of 2000." *Criminal Justice, 5,* 407–430.

Stolz, B. A. (2007). Interpreting the U.S. human trafficking debate through the lens of symbolic politics. *Law & Policy, 29,* 311–338.

Teitelbaum, J., Cartwright-Smith, L., & Rosenbaum, S. (2012). Translating rights into access: Language access and the Affordable Care Act. *American Journal of Law & Medicine, 38,* 348–373.

United Nations. (1966). *International Covenant on Economic, Social and Cultural Rights.* Retrieved from http://www.ohchr.org/EN/ProfessionalInterest/Pages/cescr.aspx

United Nations Economic and Social Council. (2000). *Substantive Issues Arising in the Implementation of the International Covenant on Economic, Social and Cultural Rights.* Retrieved from http://www.who.int/disasters/repo/13849_files/o/UN_human_rights.htm

United Nations Office on Drugs and Crime. (2004). *United Nations Convention against Transnational Crime and the Protocols Thereto.* Retrieved from http://www.unodc.org/documents/treaties/UNTOC/Publications/TOC%20Convention/TOCebook-e.pdf

U.S. Department of State. (n.d.). Victims of Trafficking and Violence Prevention Act of 2000. Retrieved from http://www.state.gov/j/tip/laws/61124.htm

van Dijk, P. & van Hoof, G. H. J. (1998). *Theory and practice of the European Convention on Human Rights.* Cambridge, MA: Kluwer Law International.

van Wormer, K. (2004). *Confronting oppression, restoring justice: From policy analysis to social action.* Alexandria, VA: Council on Social Work Education.

Witkin, S. L. (1998). Human rights and social work. *Social Work, 43,* 197–201.

Witness. (n.d.). *Paraguay's mental health system – update: Follow up to the legal petition before the IACHR.* Retrieved from http://www2.witness.org/index.php?option=com_rightsalert&Itemid=178&task=view&alert_id=22

Wronka, J. (2008). *Human rights and social justice: Social action and service for the helping and health professions.* Thousand Oaks, CA: Sage.

Civic Engagement and Civic Literacy Among Social Work Students: Where Do We Stand?

MARY E. HYLTON

School of Social Work, University of Nevada, Reno, Nevada, USA

Civic engagement is pivotal to the survival of the social work profession and to our historic role in shaping the social contract. Recent studies report declining rates of civic engagement and civic literacy among Americans. This article, which was presented at the Policy Conference 2.0, examines civic engagement and civic literacy among social work students at a medium-sized program in the western United States. Findings from this study indicate that these students are more likely to be engaged in volunteering and fundraising than in politically oriented activities. Results suggest that understanding of government and democratic processes lead to more civic engagement.

Although social work does not stand as the sole proprietor of the welfare state, arguably few other professions have as much of an interest in it as do we. Since the inception of the profession, social workers have been pivotal in articulating how our social contract will be realized in relation to those who are most vulnerable within society. The policy innovations for which the profession has fought have not only become the foundation of the welfare state but also the bread and butter for most social workers today. As Hoefer (2010, p. 161) states, "... social workers have not only an ethical duty to know how to advocate well, but also a strong self-interest in being able to persuade decision makers." Our willingness and ability to engage civically and to advocate politically is pivotal not only to ensuring the well-being of all in our society, but also to the profession's own survival.

History illustrates the symbiotic relationship between the profession and the welfare state. The profession of social work did not simply develop alongside the modern welfare state. From the reformers of the Progressive Era and the social work leaders who shaped the New Deal and Social Security act to today's policy practitioners, social workers have pushed, prodded, battled, and joined policymakers to arrive at the policies and programs that make-up our modern welfare state. Social workers reflect our society's commitment, albeit reluctant, to provide opportunities and care to those who are most disadvantaged. However, within the past 20 years, social work's relationship with the welfare state in particular and policymaking in general has been questioned (Fisher, Weedman, Alex, & Stout, 2001; Ritter, 2008). It has been suggested that the profession is abandoning its role as policy advocate and instead is placing increasing emphasis on issues of concern to direct, clinical practice (Specht & Courtney, 1994).

The profession has arrived at a crucial moment in regard to our role in shaping society's understanding of the social contract. Will the profession continue its role in advocating for a social contract inclusive of and attentive to the needs of all? Will it do so effectively in an era of globalization and the increased influence of money on policymaking? (Reich, 2012) Adding to the complexity of this moment, is the emergence of a new generation of social workers who have mostly come of age in an era of cutbacks, privatization, declining rates of public engagement in and understanding of the social contract, and a professional context in which advocacy has arguably assumed a backseat. As those social workers who were educated during the last major reform era, e.g., the 1960s, retire, what role will social work play in relation to articulating the needs of the most vulnerable in the coming decades? How prepared and interested is this new generation of social workers for engaging in the work of shaping the welfare state? This study examines the civic engagement of a sample of social work students enrolled in a medium-sized social work program in the western United States. Civic engagement is an important indicator of involvement and belief in a social contract. In addition, this study examines the civic literacy of these students as a possible means of increasing rates of civic engagement.

LITERATURE REVIEW

Civic Engagement

> For a nation whose history begins with *We The People* it seems self evident that citizen engagement matters. . . . To sustain itself, to meet challenges and thrive, democracy demands much from its citizens. (Keeter, Zukin, Andolina, & Jenkins, 2002, p. 4)

Civic engagement is an important indicator of our commitment to and involvement with the social contract. Civic engagement refers to those activities through which we demonstrate our sense of belonging to a larger social order as well as our understanding of a mutuality of responsibility for the common good. "Civic behavior increases awareness of collective interests and breaks down walls of insularity, leading to greater understanding and trust" (Keeter, Zukin, Andolina, & Jenkins, 2002, p. 4). Contrary to the beliefs of some political conservatives, civic engagement doesn't only encompass the Tocquelillian ideal of voluntary associations supplanting a centralized bureaucratic government (Skocpol, 1997). It also includes democratic efforts to engage with government and, in the case of social work, engagement with the purpose of building a fair and just society. Specifically, civic engagement encompasses participation in both civic and political endeavors. Civic activities include activities such as volunteering, voluntary membership, community problem solving, and charitable fundraising. Political activities include activities such as voting, campaigning, boycotting, contacting media outlets, contacting public officials, testifying, signing petitions, political canvassing, and participating in protests (Keeter, Zukin, Andolina, & Jenkins, 2002).

Recent reports raise serious concerns about civic engagement among the general U.S. population (Association of American Colleges and Universities (AACU), 2012; Keeter et al., 2002; Putnam, 2001). In particular, indicators of our engagement in political activities illustrate a decline in America's civic life. In 2007, the United States ranked 139th in voter participation of 172 world democracies (AACU, 2012). During the 2010 congressional elections, only 37% of eligible Americans voted (U.S. Census Bureau, 2012). Of particular concern, political participation in younger generations appears to be declining. Keeter, et al. (2002) report that fewer than a quarter of eligible voters younger than age 24 report "always voting" and that voter turnout among young people has declined by nearly 15 percentage points over the past four decades. These authors also found that only 38% of young people (ages 15–25) believed that citizenship comes with special obligations, compared to 48% of people in Generation X and 60% of baby boomers. In response to these indicators, the Obama administration commissioned a report on civic learning and democratic engagement within U.S. colleges and universities. This report described the state of American civic life as "anemic" (AACU, 2012). The authors report that half of all U.S. states no longer require civics education for high school graduation and only a third of college and university students felt that their civic engagement was strengthened by postsecondary education (AACU, 2012).

Given the apparent decline in many forms of civic engagement within the last few decades, researchers have sought to identify variables that could increase rates of civic involvement among Americans. Within the general population, increased civic engagement has been correlated with the presence of children under age 18 in the home (Caputo, 2010), education, socioeconomic status (Hauser, 2000; Keeter et al., 2002), race/ethnicity, and parental volunteerism (Caputo, 2010; Keeter et al., 2002). Additionally, Portney and O'Leary (2007, p. 5) found that college students were "almost twice as likely to be very involved as non-college young people."

Social Work and Civic Engagement

More than 20 years ago, Specht and Courtney (1994) suggested that the social work profession was abandoning its historical role as policy advocate in favor of clinical practice. Unfortunately, the move away from policy advocacy in favor of clinical practice can be seen in the number of programs offering macro concentrations. As of 2013, 25% of Council on Social Work Education (CSWE) accredited MSW programs offered concentrations in community organization and 11.6% offered concentrations in social policy (Council on Social Work Education, 2013). By contrast, over 56% of MSW programs offered clinical/direct practice concentrations. Clinical/direct practice concentrations were also overwhelmingly the most popular among students, with enrollments 6 to 12 times higher than the social policy and community organization concentrations respectively (CSWE, 2013).

Despite concerns regarding the profession's move away from political advocacy, recent studies show that social workers fare better than the general population in relation to civic engagement (Mary, 2002; Ritter, 2008; Rome & Hoechstetter, 2010). Social workers report high levels of voting, keeping up on the news, knowing their elected representatives, and encouraging others to vote (Rome & Hoechstetter, 2010). However, Ritter (2008) found that although rates of involvement were above those reported in studies of the general U.S. population, over half of licensed social workers could be characterized as "inactive" politically. Similarly, Rome and Hoechstetter (2010) found that 53% of NASW members who responded to their survey could be characterized as falling in the "low" range of political activity

As indicated earlier, civic engagement can be reflected in a variety of activities. While distinct in their nature, civic activities and political activities frequently overlap as people involved with civic activities often seek to push their causes' interests in the political realm. Both forms have historically played a role in implementing and shaping our social contract and the resulting welfare state (Skocpol, 1997). To date, much of the research on civic engagement among social workers has focused largely on involvement in political activities with little attention paid to involvement in civic activities. Therefore, little is known about social workers current rates of involvement civic activities outside of typical job duties. However, in studies of political participation, social workers are more likely to engage in activities that can be characterized as "passive," or more conventional and less confrontational (Ritter, 2008; Rome & Hoechstetter, 2010). In contrast, they are less likely to engage in more confrontational forms of advocacy. For example, social workers are less likely to engage in legislative testimony, rallies, marches, demonstrations, campaigning, donating to candidates, or to have contacted the media or their legislators (Rome & Hoechstetter, 2010).

Prior studies have illuminated several variables that are related to political participation among social workers. For example, type of employment appears to be related to political participation. Macro practitioners and public human service employees have been found to be more politically active than clinical social workers or those working for for-profit organizations (Mary, 2002; Rome & Hoechstetter, 2010). Interestingly, Rome and Hoechstetter (2010) found little difference between BSW and MSW practitioners. However, these authors report that those social workers with a PhD did have higher levels of political participation than did social workers with bachelors or masters degrees. These authors also found that social workers who were older reported more political participation than younger workers or social workers with fewer years of practice experience. This finding mirrors trends in the general population (Caputo, 2010).

Civic Literacy

> A people's capacity to govern itself democratically is . . . proportionate to the degree of its understanding of the structure and functioning of the whole social body. (Koestler, 1941, p. 168)

Civic literacy has been cited as being positively related to civic engagement (Center for Information and Research on Civic Learning and Engagement (CIRCLE), 2013; Hauser, 2000). The Center for Information and Research on Civic Learning and Engagement (CIRCLE, 2013, p. 5) demonstrated the relationship between civic engagement and civic literacy when they found that ". . . young people who do not vote lag far behind young voters in their political knowledge." While there is still some disagreement as to what civic literacy entails, most researchers agree that it includes an understanding of the democratic process and ". . . an ability to follow political events" (Lyons, Jaeger, * Wolak, 2012, p. 185). Civic literacy requires a basic understanding of the structure and functioning of government as well as the political process through which decisions are shaped. As the previous definition implies, it also requires the ability to understand and critically analyze current policy issues.

Unfortunately, recent studies have found low rates of civic literacy among Americans (CIRCLE, 2013; U.S. Department of Education, Institute of Education Sciences, National Center for Education Statistics (NCES), 2011). For example, a 2006/2007 study found the average score on a civics exam among 14,000 college seniors to be in the failing range (AACU, 2012).

Furthermore, in 2012 only 34% of adults could identify the majority party in the U.S. House of Representatives (Pew Research Center for the People & the Press, 2012). The lack of knowledge about our national democracy is concerning, and there is even less understanding of state-level government. In a 1992 study, only 54% of respondents could correctly identify whether their state had a state constitution (Lyons, Jaeger, & Wolack, 2012). In the same study, 44% could not name one branch of state government.

While Americans on a whole evidence declining civic literacy, some groups fare better than others in relation to their understanding of political and democratic processes. Scores on the National Assessment of Educational Progress indicate that students from affluent families score higher than do their classmates from low-income families (NCES, 2011). Furthermore, "Black, Hispanic and American Indian/Alaskan Native" students scored lower than did "white" students, with students identified as "black" scoring, on average, 24 to 30 points lower than students identified as "white." Kahne and Middaugh (2008, p. 5) found that "students who are more academically successful or white and those with parents of higher socioeconomic status receive more classroom-based civic learning opportunities." These disparities are particularly concerning when the relationship between civic literacy and engagement is considered. Lower civic literacy could hamper the ability of members of historically disenfranchised or oppressed groups to effectively challenge oppressive social and economic structures.

Within social work, little attention has been paid to civic literacy. Ritter (2008) included seven questions related to civic literacy in her survey of licensed social workers and found that respondents scored "fairly well." Despite the overall positive scores on these questions, only 46% of respondents could identify their state's U.S. senators and only 53% knew that it took a two-thirds majority to override a presidential veto. Given the overall decline in civic literacy over the last few decades (AACU, 2012; CIRCLE, 2012), it is important to continue to examine the political and civic knowledge of social workers, particularly those just entering the profession. To date, there have been no published studies that seek to examine the relationship between civic literacy and civic engagement among social work students.

METHODS

This study employed an online survey to examine the rates of civic engagement and civic literacy among bachelor of social work (BSW) and master of social work (MSW) students enrolled in a medium-sized public university in the western United States. The online survey included 20 civic literacy questions, the Civic Engagement Quiz (CIRCLE, n.d.) and demographic questions. Based upon previous findings regarding the effects of political knowledge on civic engagement (CIRCLE, 2013; Hauser, 2000), it was hypothesized that civic literacy would have a positive relationship with civic engagement. In particular, it was hypothesized that civic literacy would be positively related to two of the three civic engagement subscales: political voice and electoral activities.

The social work sample included within this study was drawn from a larger sample of students from all majors across campus. An invitation to participate in the study as well as a link to the survey was sent via e-mail to a random sample of undergraduate and graduate students at the university during the spring 2014 semester. In addition, students enrolled in select social work classes were sent recruitment e-mails and a link to the study. To ensure that students of varying ages and social work experience were included in the study, six social work classes representative of each educational level (e.g., freshman, junior, senior, foundation MSW, and concentration MSW) were selected for recruitment. These six courses included introduction to social work; social work and social welfare; human behavior and the social environment at both the junior and MSW foundation levels; macro social work methods at the senior level; and program evaluation at the MSW concentration level. Three follow-up e-mails were sent during the semester. Only students who indicated that they were majoring in social work are included in the results reported in this article.

The civic literacy measure included twenty multiple-choice questions, of which 15 were drawn from the Civics Assessment Database compiled by the Educational Commission of the States (Educational Commission of the States [ECS], 2014). A combination of questions from both the eighth grade and twelfth grade assessments was used in this study. These questions focused largely on principles of American democracy and constitutional issues. In addition, four questions about national political leadership were asked to ascertain students' knowledge of current political functioning. All of the questions were multiple choice. In addition to looking at items individually, overall scores on the civic literacy questions were calculated by adding the number of correct answers provided by individual respondents.

The Civic Engagement Quiz is a 26-item measure of civic engagement developed by researchers at the Center for Information & Research on Civic Learning and Engagement (CIRCLE, n.d.) using indicators outlined by Keeter and colleagues (2002). This instrument has three subscales reflecting different dimensions of civic engagement, including civic activities, electoral activities, and political voice. Civic activities include voluntary memberships, volunteering and raising money for charitable causes. Electoral activities included activities centered on voting and influencing election outcomes. Finally, political voice encompasses activities that seek to influence policymaking, such as testifying, signing petitions, or contacting public officials. On all of the items, respondents indicate their involvement by answering yes or no.

Just over 100 social work students completed the survey ($n = 101$). The majority of these surveys were completed by students in the BSW program (83%), with a smaller number being completed by students in the MSW program (17%). Of those in the BSW program the majority of respondents identified as being juniors (48%) or seniors (45%) with significantly fewer freshmen or sophomores (7% total). Not surprisingly, 92% of respondents identified as female and eight% identified as male. These numbers were representative of the gender distribution of both programs. Respondents were asked to identify their race or ethnicity. Sixty-four percent of the sample identified as Caucasian, 17% as Latino or Hispanic, 4% as African American, 2% as Native American or American Indian, and 5% as Asian American. Based on these numbers, Latino students were underrepresented in the sample, as they constitute approximately 30% of the BSW student population.

RESULTS

All respondents reported involvement in civic endeavors. On average, respondents reported having been involved in 11 civic engagement activities during their lifetimes. Current and past involvement in civic endeavors among this sample of social work students ranged from 3 to 21 out of a possible 24 activities. However, levels of participation varied significantly based upon the nature of the activities. Civic activities had the highest reported involvement with on average six activities out of a possible nine, followed in order by political voice and electoral activities. Students were most likely to have volunteered with health and human services (76%) and youth services (78%) as well as to have helped raise money for nonprofit organizations (77%). They were least likely to have volunteered in relation to environmental causes (28%). Further, 40% of the students reported not currently belonging to any voluntary associations, groups, clubs, etc. Table 1 provides the percentage of student involvement in all 24 indicators of civic engagement.

Students reported involvement in an average of 3.9 out of nine political voice activities. Overall, students reported higher rates of involvement in political voice activities that required less investment of time/effort (see Table 1). For example, students were more likely to sign petitions either electronic or written (70% and 68% respectively) but less likely to have contacted an elected official (38%) or a media outlet (18% newspaper and 6% broadcast media). They were more likely to boycott or support companies (75% and 76% respectively). In addition, only 31% had participated in a march or protest.

By contrast, electoral activities had the lowest rate of involvement at an average of 1.3 out of six. Nearly 40% of students reported no engagement either current or previously in electoral activities (other than irregular

TABLE 1 Percentage of Students Involved in Civic Engagement Activities

	Involved
Civic Activities	
Have you volunteered or done any voluntary community services for no pay?	99%
Have you volunteered for an organization for youth, children or education?	79%
Have you volunteered with a civic or community organization involved in health or social services?	77%
Besides donating money, have you ever done anything else to help raise money for a charitable cause?	77%
Have you ever worked together with someone or some group to solve a problem in the community where you live?	70%
Have you personally walked, ran or bicycled for a charitable cause?	66%
Do you currently belong to any voluntary groups, clubs or associations?	61%
Have you volunteered with a religious group?	55%
Have you volunteered with an environmental organization?	28%
Political Voice	
Have you bought something because you have liked the social or political values of the company that produces or provides it?	76%
Have you ever NOT bought something from a certain company because you disagree with the social or political values of the company that produces it?	75%
Shave you ever signed an email petition about a social or political issue?	70%
Have you ever signed a written petition about a political or social issue?	68%
Have you ever contacted or visited a public official at any level of government to express your opinion?	38%
Have you ever taken part in a protest, march or demonstration?	32%
Have you contacted a newspaper or magazine to express your opinion?	18%
Have you worked as a canvasser going door to door for a political or social group or candidate?	13%
Have you contacted broadcast media to express your opinion?	6%
Electoral Activities	
We know that most people don't vote in all elections. Do you vote in both national and local elections?	31%[a]
Do you wear a campaign button, put a sticker on your car, or place a sign in front of your house?	33%
When there is an election taking place, do you try to convince people to vote for or against one of the parties or candidates, or not?	32%
Have you volunteered for a political organization or candidate running for office?	22%
Have you ever given money to a candidate, political party, or organization that supported candidates?	12%

Note. N = 101. All percentages have been rounded.
[a]Participants were able to select "always," "usually" or "never" in response to this question. Only the "always" answers were included in the "Yes" column to indicate regular voting.
[b]Responses of "never" are reported in the "no" column.

voting). Of particular concern, only 31% of students reported always voting in national or local elections, while 10% reported never voting. The remaining 59% of the sample reported "usually" voting (see Table 1). Relatedly, 22% of students reported not being registered to vote at their current residence. The majority reported that they do not attempt to persuade others or display campaign material in relation to candidates or election issues (see Table 1). Furthermore, fewer than a quarter (22%) of the students reported volunteering for political organizations or campaigns and even fewer have canvased in relation to campaigns (13%). Finally, students were very unlikely to have donated money to campaigns (16%).

Scores on the civic literacy measure illustrated the variance in knowledge among social work students about government and the U.S. political process. Scores ranged from 4 to 20 out of a possible 20. The average score was 14.63 or a C-. While nearly a quarter of the students scored in what could be classified as the "A" range, 90% or higher, more than a third of the students scored in the "D" range, 69% or lower. On several items, students showed a near uniform understanding. For example, the majority of the students could identify the three branches of the federal government and were able to identify the first 10 amendments to the Constitution as being the Bill of Rights (see Table 2). However, nearly half of the students were unable to answer correctly four of the questions. For example, 45% of respondents were not able to identify an example of state-federal cooperation and 46% did not know which branch of government has the power to tax. Students scored particularly poorly on three of the four questions about current political leadership. Forty-four percent were not able to identify the current Speaker of the House and 35% did not know which party currently holds the majority in the House. Similarly, 22% were not able to identify the current Senate Majority Leader, (who also served as one of the two U.S. Senators from the state in which the University is located). Finally, 17% could not identify their own current U.S. Senators.

A Pearson correlation was computed to assess the relationship between rates of civic engagement and civic literacy. There was a significant, moderate relationship ($r = .356$, $n = 101$, $p = .000$), between involvement in civic engagement activities and civic literacy scores, thereby disproving the null hypothesis that the two variables are not related. When looking at the relationship between civic literacy and the three types of civic engagement activities specifically, only two of the types showed a significant relationship. There was a weak relationship between electoral activities and civic literacy ($r = .258$, $n = 101$, $p = .009$). There was a moderate relationship between political voice activities and civic literacy ($r = .387$, $n = 101$, $p = .000$). These findings support the hypotheses that civic literacy is related to political participation.

TABLE 2 Percentage of Correct Reponses on Civic Literacy Questions

	Correct
What are the three branches of the national government of the United States?	96%
Soon after the Constitution of the United States was approved, 10 amendments were added to it. These 10 amendments are known as the	95%
How did women in the United States get the right to vote?	86%
The ability of the United States Supreme Court to declare an act of Congress, or an act of the President, unconstitutional is an example of	85%
Identify the two Senators who currently represent Nevada in the United States Senate.	82%
According to the United States constitution, which of the following has the power to declare war?	81%
How many representatives does each state have in the United States House of Representatives?	75%
Which party holds the majority in the United States Senate?	77%
The primary purpose of the Bill of Rights was to	76%
Who is the current Majority Leader within the United States Senate?	74%
How many Senators does each state have in the United States Senate?	73%
Which of these principles of government is demonstrated when the governor of a state vetoes a bill?	73%
What is the primary source of money to operate the national government?	70%
Which of these bodies has the authority to make laws?	69%
In a democratic political system, which of the following ought to govern the country?	68%
Which party holds the majority of members in the United States House of Representatives?	64%
The number of electoral votes each state is allotted is based on the state's . . . ?	59%
Who is the current Speaker of the United States House of Representatives?	56%
Under the United States Constitution, the power to tax belongs to the . . . ?	54%
Which of the following activities is an example of cooperation between state and national governments?	54%

Note. N = 101. All percentages have been rounded.

T-tests were conducted to compare rates of civic engagement and civic literacy between BSW and MSW students. There was no significant difference in rates of civic engagement based upon enrollment in either the BSW or MSW programs ($df = 99$, $t = 1.53$, $p = .127$). However, there was a significant difference in civic literacy scores between BSW and MSW students ($df = 99$, $t = 2.04$, $p = .04$), with MSW students scoring on average higher ($m = 16$) than BSW students ($m = 14$). In addition, a one-way Analysis of Variance revealed no significant difference at the $p < .05$ level in rates of civic engagement based on race/ethnicity [$F(8, 92) = .841$, $p = .569$].

DISCUSSION

Students in this medium-sized social work education program reported high rates of civic engagement overall. All students reported involvement in at least one civic engagement activity, with the majority reporting involvement in multiple activities. Most of this involvement occurred in the nonpolitical domain of civic activities. For example, nearly all of the students engaged in some form of volunteerism. Arguably, those volunteer activities with the highest rates of involvement mirror the traditional realm of social services. Students were most likely to have volunteered with organizations associated with health, youth, and educational services as well as in charitable fundraising activities. Voluntarily giving time to such organizations may reflect students' career interests and the service-mission of the profession. In addition, the reporting of engagement in these activities may be somewhat inflated by students whose involvement included field practicum-related activities. However, it should be noted that more than half of the students (55%) had not completed a field practicum prior to taking the survey and, therefore, would not have been able to include practicum-related activities in their reporting of civic engagement.

The minimal reporting of volunteerism with environmental organizations by these students raises questions about the recognition of a larger, more encompassing social contract. Although rarely directly related to the provision of social services, environmental issues significantly influence the well-being of society, making the work of these organizations vital to our articulation of a social contract. Furthermore, environmental hazards or problems disproportionately affect low-income communities, making such issues important targets for social work advocacy. Unfortunately, the students' lack of involvement in environmental activities could reflect a belief that their involvement or service activities do not extend beyond direct social service organizations.

Students reported lower levels of involvement in political voice and electoral activities. Within the political domain, students were more likely to be involved in those activities that involved minimal risk and minimal investment of time such as signing petitions and boycotting or supporting companies. They were least likely to have worked as political canvassers, to have contacted a public official, to have given money to support a candidate, or to have contacted the broadcast media to express an opinion on a political issue. This pattern of involvement again raises questions about how this group of social work students understands their role in shaping the social contract or the social welfare state. While participation in petitions and boycotts evidences some willingness to support movements to change social institutions, the minimal levels of involvement in higher risk activities illustrates a weak political voice and, therefore, a minimal role in shaping the social welfare state.

The finding that nearly 40% of the students reported no involvement in electoral activities is especially concerning. Only 32% of these students report always voting and only slightly more than a third of students try to influence people to vote for a particular candidate or party during an election. These findings mirror the trend of declining political involvement among younger generations (Keeter et al., 2002). Declining involvement in political voice and electoral activities directly affects the profession's role in shaping a just social contract. Therefore, further study of social work students' involvement in these activities is needed to determine if this trend is evident in larger, more representative samples. Future studies should address not just rates of involvement but motivations or barriers to involvement. For example, why are social work students reluctant to engage in electoral activities specifically or in the political arena in general? Identifying barriers to involvement may assist social work educators in providing learning opportunities that foster the political voice of students.

In response to this study's question about the influence of civic literacy on civic engagement, this study did find that understanding of constitutional issues and democratic processes does play a role in the civic engagement of social work students. In particular, civic literacy leads to greater involvement in electoral and political voice-oriented activities. As students' understanding of their government increases, so do their efforts to influence the democratic process. This finding illustrates the need for greater attention to civic literacy within social work education. Unfortunately, students in this study underperformed on civic literacy. MSW students scored, on average, higher than did BSW students, yet more than a third of all of the students scored a 69% or lower. Too many of the students were unable to identify key political leaders and a sizable number could not answer the two questions related to federal revenue. Once again, further study with larger, multi-site samples are needed to ascertain whether these patterns of civic literacy are widespread.

Given the lower rates of involvement in political voice and electoral activities, social work educators should seek to identify and implement strategies to assist their students in becoming more engaged politically. First, attention should be paid to increasing civic literacy among social work students. Social work students need a solid understanding of democratic processes/functioning in order to influence said processes. Increased emphasis on not just the products of policy but also on the intricacies of policymaking and funding at the federal, state, local and organizational levels will assist students in identifying when and how they can influence policy with the greatest effectiveness. For example, educators can organize events that introduce students to current election and legislative issues. Just as service learning and volunteer requirements facilitate student engagement in civic activities, so too might voter-registration drives, get-out-the-vote drives, legislative visits, letter-writing campaigns, public information campaigns, etc., facilitate greater involvement in political and electoral activities. In particular, legislative day events, which are sometimes referred to as "Lobby Days" or Legislative, Education, and Advocacy, e.g., LEAD Days, could provide intensive experiences that might build student interest in political voice activities (DeRigne, Rosenwald, & Naranjo, 2014). Many schools already benefit from annual social work legislative days, but those programs that do not require student participation in such events should consider developing or involving their students in such events.

Clearly, a significant limitation of this study is its lack of generalizability to other social work programs. However, as an exploratory study, the findings raise important questions for future study, including how social work students view their role in shaping the social contract. What prevents students from being engaged civically, particularly in political processes? How well do social work students understand their government and policymaking? Finally, is the relationship between civic literacy and civic engagement generalizable and, therefore, an important target for intervention? All of these questions should be addressed with larger samples pulled from social work education programs representative of diverse social and educational contexts.

CONCLUSION

Civic engagement is an important component of the profession's historic role in shaping the social contract and the resulting welfare state. Social workers' ability to define problems in macro as well as micro terms and our willingness to intervene in social issues that others are unwilling to acknowledge the profession's historic broad understanding of society's responsibility to one another and to the most vulnerable. This understanding is also reflected in our profession's commitment to social and economic justice, which is articulated clearly in the National Association of Social Workers' Code of Ethics as well as the International Federation of Social Workers' Statement of Ethical Principles. Most important, civic engagement underlies the profession's symbiotic relationship with social welfare policy. Historically, social work has played a pivotal role both in providing policy solutions and in advocating for just social policies to address significant social problems within our society.

While the findings of this study cannot be generalized to all social work students, several conclusions can be reached in relation to civic engagement and the profession's continuing role in the welfare state. First, social work students in this sample were less active in political and electoral activities than they were in civic activities such as charitable fundraising and volunteering. This finding reflects a possible narrowing of how the profession's role in the welfare state is understood. Second, the finding that students were less likely to engage in active, high-risk forms of political advocacy mirrors findings of other studies in regard to social workers' political involvement (Rome

& Hoechstetter, 2010; Ritter, 2008). This supports the concern that the next generation of social workers may take a more passive role within the welfare state and may not be prepared to engage fully in shaping this social institution. Finally, the finding that civic engagement, in particular engagement in political voice and electoral activities, is related to civic literacy provides a potential path for addressing the aforementioned concerns.

Social work educators need to ensure that the next generation of social workers (e.g., those who are today's students) will continue the profession's role in shaping the welfare state. To do so, we need to ensure that students are engaged civically. In particular, we need to ensure that students are willing and prepared to engage in the democratic processes that shape our social contract. Without this engagement, social work educators risk educating students to be good agency practitioners, but not good citizens. We risk losing our professional role, not just as deliverers of social welfare programs, but as the architects of the welfare state.

REFERENCES

The Association of American Colleges and Universities. (2012). *A crucible moment: College learning & democracy's future*. Retrieved from http://www.aacu.org/civiclearning/crucible

Caputo, R. K. (2010). Family characteristics, public program participation and civic engagement. *Journal of Sociology & Social Welfare, 37*(2), 35–61.

Center for Information and Research on Civic Learning and Engagement. (n.d.). Civic engagement quiz. Retrieved from CIRCLE's Tools for Practice http://www.civicyouth.org/PopUps/Final_Civic_Inds_Quiz_2006.pdf

Center for Information and Research on Civic Learning and Engagement. (2013). Fact sheet: What do young adults know about politics? Evidence from a national survey conducted after the 2012 election. Retrieved from http://www.civicyouth.org/wp-content/uploads/2013/01/What-Young-Adults-Know-Fact-Sheet-20131.pdf

Council on Social Work Education. (2013). 2013 statistics on social work education in the United States. Retrieved from http://www.cswe.org/CentersInitiatives/DataStatistics/ProgramData/74475.aspx

DeRigne, L., Rosenwald, M., & Naranjo, F. (2014). Legislative advocacy and social work education: Models and new strategies. *Journal of Policy Practice, 13*(4), 316–327.

Educational Commission of the States. (2014). Resources to assess student civic competencies and school climate. Retrieved from http://www.ecs.org/Qna/splash_new.asp

Fisher, R., Weedman, A., Alex, G., & Stout, K. D. (2001). Graduate education for social change: A study of political social workers. *Journal of Community Practice, 9*(4), 43–64.

Hauser, S. M. (2000). Education, ability, and civic engagement in the contemporary United States. *Social Sciences Research, 29*, 556–582. doi:10.1006/ssre.2000.0681

Hoefer, R. (2010). Introduction: Contemporary research on social work advocacy and policy practice. *Journal of Policy Practice, 9*(3-4), 161–163. doi:10.1080/15588742.2010.489107

Kahne, J., & Middaugh, E. (2008). Democracy for some: The civic opportunity gap in high school (CIRCLE Working Paper 59). Retrieved from The Center for Information and Research on Civic Learning and Engagement http://www.civicyouth.org/PopUps/WorkingPapers/WP59Kahne.pdf

Keeter, S., Zukin, C., Andolina, M., & Jenkins, K. (2002). The civic and political health of the nation: A generational portrait. Retrieved from The Center for Information and Research on Civic Learning and Civic Engagement http://files.eric.ed.gov/fulltext/ED498892.pdf

Koestler, A. (1941). *Darkness at noon*. New York, NY: MacMillan Company.

Lyons, J., Jaeger, W. P., & Wolak, J. (2012). The roots of citizens' knowledge of state politics. *State Politics & Policy Quarterly, 13*(2)c, 183–202. doi:10.1177/1532440012464878

Mary, N. L. (2002). Political activism of social work educators. *Journal of Community Practice, 9*(4), 1–20.

Pew Research Center for the People & the Press. (2012). *Pew Research Center for the People* & the Press *Political Knowledge Survey, July, 2012*. Retrieved from http://www.people-press.org/question-search/?qid=1815615&pid=51&ccid=50

Portney, K. E. & O'Leary, L. (2007). *Civic and political engagement of America's youth: A report from the Tisch College "National Survey of civic and political engagement of young people."* Retrieved from Tufts University, Tisch College of Citizenship and Public Service http://activecitizen.tufts.edu/wp-content/uploads/FinalReport1.pdf

Putnam, R. D. (2001). Civic disengagement in contemporary America. *Government and Opposition, 36*(2), 135–156. doi:10.1111/1477-7053.00059

Reich, R. (2012). *Beyond outrage: What has gone wrong with our economy and our democracy, and how to fix it*. New York, NY: Vintage.

Ritter, J. (2008). Evaluating the political participation of licensed social workers in the new millennium. *Journal of Policy Practice, 6*(4), 61–78. doi:10.1300/J508v06n04_05

Rome, S. H., & Hoechstetter, S. (2010). Social work and civic engagement: The political participation of professional social workers. *Journal of Sociology & Social Welfare, 37*(3), 107–129.

Skocpol, T. (1997). The Tocqueville problem: Civic engagement in American democracy, *Social Science History, 21*(4), 455–479.

Specht, H., & Courtney, M. (1994). *Unfaithful angels: How social work has abandoned its mission*. New York, NY: The Free Press.

U.S. Census Bureau. (2012). *Voting and registration in the election of November 2010*. Retrieved from http://www.census.gov/hhes/www/socdemo/voting/publications/p20/2010/tables.html

U.S. Department of Education, Institute of Education Sciences, National Center for Education Statistics. (2011). *The Nation's report card: Civics 2010 a national assessment of educational progress at grades 4, 8, and 12*. Retrieved from National Center for Education http://nces.ed.gov/nationsreportcard/pdf/main2010/2011466.pdf

Solving Current Social Challenges: Engaging Undergraduates in Policy Practice

MARGARET SHERRADEN
School of Social Work, University of Missouri-St. Louis, and Center for Social Development, Washington University, St. Louis, Missouri, USA

BAORONG GUO
School of Social Work, University of Missouri-St. Louis, and Center for Social Development, Washington University, St. Louis, Missouri

CHRISTINE UMBERTINO
Brown School of Social Work, Washington University, St. Louis, Missouri

This article explores an innovation in teaching policy practice at the undergraduate level. It analyzes an experiential learning model that uses current social challenges as a compelling way to generate student learning about policy practice. Over the course of the semester, students examine antecedents, current issues, and potential solutions to a contemporary social issue through a series of assignments that build knowledge and skills and link the topic to larger social policy concerns. Using quantitative and qualitative evidence from seven semesters, the article explores benefits and challenges of this approach to teaching, and derives lessons for social work education.

"I'm starting to realize policy is social work and social work is policy" (BSW student)

Historically, social workers have played key roles in shaping social policies to address the needs of vulnerable populations (American Academy of Social Work and Social Welfare, 2013). Scholars underscore the essential role of policy practice in social work (Abramovitz, 1993; Cummins, Byers, & Pedrick, 2011; Figueira-McDonough, 1993; Hoefer, 2006; Iatridis, 1995; Jansson, 2010; Rocha, 2007; Wyers, 1990). Unfortunately, over the past 50 years, policy practice by social workers has taken a backseat to clinical practice (Rothman, 2012; Specht & Courtney, 1994). As Alice Johnson asked 10 years ago, "social work is standing on the legacy of Jane Addams, but are we sitting on the sidelines?" (2004).

Jack Rothman (2012, p. 17) concludes in a recent report on macro practice, that "the pattern of intervention modes in social work is clearly out of balance, with community and societal approaches to human and social development in the shadow." In a follow-up commentary, Rothman and Terri Mizrahi (2014, p. 1), implore the profession to "recalibrate the imbalance between micro and macro practice." An important element of such a "recalibration" is effective teaching of policy practice in social work.

What is policy practice? According to the profession's largest association, policy practice "encompasses professional efforts to influence the development, enactment, implementation, modification, or assessment of social policies, primarily to ensure social justice and equal access to basic social goods" (NASW, 2011, p. 330; see also, Clark, 2007; Social Work Policy Institute, 2012). The Council on Social Work Education (2008), which oversees professional social work education, states that one of the 10 core competencies common to all of social practice is advancing human rights and social and economic justice through understanding the forms and mechanisms of oppression and discrimination and applying strategies of advocacy and social change that advance social and economic justice (CSWE, 2008). Similarly, the NASW Code of Ethics (2008) states that:

> Social workers should engage in social and political action that seeks to ensure that all people have equal access to the resources, employment, services, and opportunities they require to meet their basic human needs and to develop fully. Social workers should be aware of the impact of the political arena on practice and should advocate for changes in policy and legislation to improve social conditions in order to meet basic human needs and promote social justice. (Section 6.04)

From an international perspective, policy is considered a core purpose of social work. According to the Global Standards for Social Work Education and Training adopted by the International Association of Schools of Social Work and the International Federation of Social Workers, social workers should "Engage in social and political action to impact social policy and economic development . . ." and core curricular standards should include, "Knowledge of social welfare policies (or lack thereof), services and laws at local, national and/or regional/ international levels, and the roles of social work in policy planning, implementation, evaluation and in social change processes" (Sewpaul & Jones, 2004).

These mandates support teaching that enables social work students to make connections between direct service and policy practice, and prepares them to influence social policy. This article identifies challenges to effective teaching of policy practice at the undergraduate level. It underscores advantages of experiential learning models in teaching policy practice, and analyzes a promising experiential model for teaching policy practice.

While incorporating elements of experiential learning in teaching policy is not completely new, documentation of its effectiveness is rare in the existing literature, especially in undergraduate teaching. There are two main reasons for this. First, from a practical point of view, empirical evaluation seems far less urgent than exploring new teaching methods to stimulate students' interest in policy practice. Second, from a technical perspective, empirical evaluation can be very challenging not only because it involves systematic methods to collect and analyze data over a long time, but also because such evaluation could be questioned due to small samples and other issues. Nonetheless, we believe it is important to evaluate the use of experiential learning in teaching policy practice given its growing popularity. This study is one of the first efforts in this direction. The study presents quantitative and qualitative evidence from seven semesters of the class offered at the upper undergraduate level at a large urban university. As discussions of teaching policy practice are on the rise, it is important to bring evidence to such discussions and inform social work educators of the benefits and challenges of this approach to teaching policy practice in social work.

TEACHING POLICY PRACTICE IN SOCIAL WORK

Instructors often struggle to make policy relevant to social work students (Fisher & Corciullo, 2011). They confront what scholars have found is a preference for direct practice or psychotherapeutic practice over policy development and engagement in social action (Abell & McDonell, 1990; Bogo, Raphael, & Roberts; 1993, Butler, 1990, 1992; Rubin, Johnson, & DeWeaver, 1986). Studies also reveal students' preference for direct practice persists from matriculation through graduation (Butler, 1990; Rubin & Johnson, 1984). As a result, students resist policy practice with the rationale, "I won't ever have to use this; I want to help *people*" (Rothman, 2011; Rubin & Johnson, 1984; Weiss, Gal, Cnaan, & Maglajlic, 2002; Weiss, Gal, & Dixon, 2003).

Historically, Walz and Groz (1991) identify a shift in the profession they call "middle classization," which led from a focus on the poor to a focus on the family. Hymans (2000) states this mission shift may be responsible for students' lack of interest in policy practice. He posits that, instead of a burning desire to "change the world" and create equal opportunity through policy change, the majority of students want to learn clinical skills to work with targeted vulnerable groups, including at-risk youth, dysfunctional families, or abused children (Hymans 2000). Trend reports from CSWE and NASW confirm that micro or clinical concentrations and specializations eclipse other specializations (2012, www.cswe.org; see also Whitaker & Arrington, 2008).

Student preference for direct practice, as well as perceptions that policy content lacks direct relevance to their chosen field challenge academics to link policy and practice (Linhorst 2002; Rocha 2000; Rocha & Johnson 1997). Strategies include additional courses with a macro focus, policy research, and policy analysis, as well as continuing education on current policies and policy advocacy (Freeman, 1996; Linhorst, 2002).

Finally, as other professions have taken up policy practice, some students interested in policy, who may once have considered social work, go elsewhere. The Association for Public Policy Analysis and Management (APPAM) reports that in the past 50 years—during the period that social work has retreated from policy practice—several public policy degrees have emerged, including Master of Public Policy, Master of Public Service, and Master of Science in Public Policy and Management (www.appam.org). Other human service professions, such as public health and education, also have developed public policy arms.

EXPERIENTIAL LEARNING: FROM SOCIAL POLICY TO POLICY PRACTICE

Despite these trends, social work can renew its strength in policy through enhanced teaching—using experiential learning to engage students. Research into the learning process suggests that traditional, didactic, teacher-focused instruction, while efficient in many ways and appropriate for certain subjects, is limited and non-effective in others. Lecture-based pedagogy works well with motivated students who can relate personally to the course content; however, it is a poor way to engage reluctant learners, including many social work students in foundation policy classes.

Experiential, student-focused, and active learning addresses some of the pitfalls of traditional lecture methods for teaching policy practice. Experiential learning is founded in the work of John Dewey, who believed education served a social purpose in helping people become engaged members of society. Unlike didactic teaching styles, Dewey advocated for educational environments in which students become equal, valued, and responsible participants (Dewey, 1938). He believed that students learn when teaching methods stimulate thinking, reflection, exploration, and experience. New research in neuroscience suggests that elements of experiential learning activate regions of the brain that assist in learning (Zull, 2004).

Expanding on Dewey's work, Kolb and Kolb (2008) proposed a model that posits learning is a continuous cycle of: (1) concrete experience, (2) abstract conceptualization, (3) reflective observation, and (4) active experimentation. Social services professionals, such as social workers tend to learn best in an environment, according to the Kolbs:

> that calls for the generation of ideas (such as a "brainstorming" session), have broad cultural interests, like to gather information, are interested in people, tend to be imaginative and emotional, prefer to work in groups, [and] listen with an open mind and receive personalized feedback. (Kolb & Kolb, 2008, p. 10)

Reflecting these insights, experiential teaching methods have gained adherents in social policy instruction. Rocha and Johnson (1997) and Rocha (2000) emphasize the importance of making social policy relevant to field experiences. Idit Weiss, John Gal, and Joseph Katan (2006, p. 796) state that "active learning, employing experiential learning" and student-focused techniques may be more effective. Student-centered approaches to teaching, such as open-group discussions, simulation games, problem-based learning, and case analyses, are more effective than lectures or traditional, instructor-centered methods (Dochy, Segers, Van Den Bossche, & Gijbels, 2003; Nuckles, 2000; Hmelo-Silver, 2004).

Scholars report on a variety of approaches for using an experiential learning approach to engage students in policy practice. Sherraden, Slosar & Sherraden (2002) describes a policy advocacy project that involved faculty, students and field instructors, that culminated in successful passage of state legislation. Gibbons & Gray (2002) discuss the Newcastle Model, in which undergraduate students select a learning activity they find relevant, and become actively involved in critical thinking and problem solving. In this way, the instructor facilitates a project on current events and social problems that spark student desire to learn and engage in social justice practice.

In Australia, social policy is an integral part of social work's four-year experience-based program social policy instruction in child protection (Gibbons & Gray, 2005). Weiss et al. (2006) propose a three-year program of study in Israeli schools of social work that requires six social policy courses, integration of policy practice in methods courses, and a concentration on policy practice (Weiss et al., 2006, p. 799). Designed to engage students in policy, it does not sidestep the question of values, suggesting that educators should be free to express their opinions in regards to policy issues (Weiss et al., 2006, p. 797–798). Most recently, Weiss-Gal and Savaya (2012) designed a three-semester seminar in policy practice for MSW students in Israel. Components included lectures, readings, guest speakers, one-on-one sessions between students and instructors, student discussion groups, and a term paper (Weiss-Gal & Savaya, 2012, p. 142). This model is unique in that it was designed to actively engage students in policy practice at their place of employment. This model could be adapted to accommodate working professionals in BSW and MSW programs.

Jansson and colleagues (2011) propose an approach they call "Practicing policy, Pursuing change, and Promoting social justice" (3P), that brings together social work students from different course sections to work on an eight-stage/multi-year advocacy project (Jansson, Fertig, Hansung, & Heidemann, 2011, p. 39). The instructor chooses a target issue based on (a) potential for meaningful impact, (b) confidence that policy change is possible, and (c) needs in the local community. Students select an element of the issue to study in depth (Jansson, et al., 2011, p. 41). Teaching challenges include timing (e.g., legislation may not coincide with the course), and lapse of activity during academic breaks (Jansson et al., 2011, p. 47).

The teaching innovations described here utilize a wide array of teaching techniques such as debates, legislative policy briefs, journal writings, role plays, media advocacy, task-force assignments, letters to the editor, service-learning projects, involvement in political campaigns, policy analysis papers, community research projects, client interviews, legislative analysis and policy papers (Social Work Policy Institute, 2012).

In sum, these teaching approaches endeavor to provide students opportunity to gain knowledge and practice skills in policy practice through combining traditional pedagogical techniques with experiential elements. Next, we turn to an approach that uses experiential education to help undergraduate social work students learn about and envision a role in policy practice. This approach is similar to Jansson's 3P model (2011), but is completed in one semester at the undergraduate level.

TEACHING POLICY PRACTICE TO UNDERGRADUATE SOCIAL WORK STUDENTS: DIVING BELOW THE HEADLINES

> "Foreclosures up 75% in 2007"—CNN (Christie, 2008)
> "Illegal Immigrants' Underground Lives Hobble their US-Born Children"—New York Times (Semple, 2011)
> "Diabetes: A local, national, and worldwide scourge"—New York Times (Kleinfield, 2006)
> "In a downturn, college strains family budgets"—New York Times (Glater, 2008)
> "Half of children killed in fires are under age 5"—USA Today (Sternberg, 2011)
> "State funding for preschool drops as Obama calls for expansion"—The Washington Post (Chandler, 2013)

Knowing that many undergraduate social work students approach social policy classes with trepidation, even resistance (Anderson & Harris, 2005;

> - House fire deaths among children (2004)
> - Household debt and bankruptcy (2005)
> - Home foreclosures (2007)
> - Type 2 diabetes (2006, 2009)
> - Student debt (2008)
> - Housing foreclosures (2010)
> - U.S. immigration (2011, 2012)
> - Early childhood care (2013)

FIGURE 1 Policy project topics in different semesters.

Hymans, 2000; Wolk, Pray, Weismiller, & Dempsey, 1996), this course focuses on a compelling social issue in the news (Figure 1). The class spends a semester studying an issue, including its antecedents, complexity, and potential solutions. At the same time, the issue is linked to the array of social policies covered in a typical foundation policy course—including social assistance, social insurance, human rights, child welfare, health, nutrition, and mental health—but the semester-long topic offers students a way to think about these larger issues.

The instructor selects the topic based on its ability to elicit connections to the key social policy issues in social work, and the likelihood that students will hear repeatedly about the topic in the media during that semester. Using the headline issue to capture students' attention, in depth exploration helps them understand the range of policies and programs that come into play in improving people's lives, and shows them how social workers engage in policy change. The semester-long project aims to make policy "come alive," and open students' minds to the many ways that policy affects well-being and life chances.

The inspiration for this approach is Eric Klinenberg's *Heat Wave: The Social Autopsy of Disaster in Chicago* (2002), in which he posits that the astronomically high death rate among older poor residents during a record-breaking hot summer was not simply an "act of God".[1] Klinenberg details the convergence of factors that made the poor, old, sick, and alone so vulnerable to heat stroke and death. Establishing cooling shelters was the city's response to the crisis, but it clearly did not solve the range of underlying issues raised in Klinenberg's book. Like Klinenberg's "autopsy," the policy course aims to analyze a particular issue in a way that opens up the world of social policy for undergraduate students.

A series of assignments build knowledge and skills over the course of the semester, addressing key aspects of policy practice. Each assignment also

---

[1] The so-called "excess death" rate (the difference between reported deaths and typical deaths for a given time period) was 739 during the week of July 14 to 20, an amount that far exceeded what would be expected even under the extreme heat of that summer (Klinenberg, 2002).

> **Part 1: What do we know about the issue?** This assignment underscore a central point: *facts and expertise matter*. In the undergraduate class, this assignment is a fact sheet.
>
> **Part 2: What are past and current policies that address this issue?** The assignment focuses on the reality that most (although not all) *policies are incremental*. In the undergraduate class, this assignment is an annotated outline of existing policies.
>
> **Part 3: What can we do to improve the situation?** This assignment underscores social workers' *roles in and responsibility for innovation and change*. In the undergraduate class, students write a policy brief that brings together what they have learned about the nature of the issue, past and current policies, with a proposal for change. The proposal can be their own or an existing proposal, but must include a rationale and justification that demonstrates understanding of the issue and social work values. Examples: Some of the students proposed bilingual educational materials for immigrant populations.
>
> **Part 4: How can we get involved?** The action part of the project *introduces policy advocacy skills*. This assignment could be writing to a legislator, writing a letter to the editor or an op-ed, or meeting with the director of an agency. In the undergraduate class, this assignment is presented in an "elevator pitch", a 3-minute persuasive speech to the class about the issue and the student's proposed solution or innovation.

FIGURE 2 Four-part policy project and deliverables.

> - The St. Louis Fire Chief discussed the anatomy of house fires.
> - A nurse from the American Diabetes Association presented "Diabetes 101."
> - Analysts from San Francisco and St. Louis Federal Reserve Boards explained the nature of the financial crisis (household debt, home foreclosures).
> - An urban planner introduced urban walkability initiatives (diabetes).
> - A lawyer from the National Consumer Law Center presented legal actions against predatory housing lenders (home foreclosures).
> - Social work advocates from Legal Aid described advocacy efforts with immigrants.
> - Missouri General Assembly members discussed their health policy proposals (diabetes).
> - A child welfare advocate, whose baby died in child care, discussed legislation she proposed (early child care).

FIGURE 3 Sample guest speakers for various policy projects.

focuses on students' learning a variety of communications skills for policy practice (see Figure 2).

Many social work students report that policy practice feels too abstract and too "big"; they find the idea intimidating. The aim of focusing on a single topic is to help them gain confidence that they can engage in policy practice. They hear from community experts, read, discuss, and debate the topic. For example, guest speakers, who reflect the multidisciplinary nature of social issues, shed light on different dimensions of each policy topic (Figure 3).

Social work students may have a more positive view of government than many Americans (Pew Research Center, 2013), but they often report a distrust of "politics" and "politicians," which they associate with policy. The policy project is the "lens" through which students learn in a tangible way how policy affects people's lives. It capitalizes on students' motivation to "help people." In the end, the policy project helps them understand that policy can do just that.

Nonetheless, even focusing on a specific topic, and learning from a series of assignments, guest speakers, films, and discussions can be challenging for students who are more comfortable with the facts of a direct service case. Policy is complex, and for some students, this can be overwhelming, especially until they have a foundational knowledge of the topic. Most students gain knowledge and confidence over the course of the semester, although some students require extra assistance.

The link between the specific policy topic and the larger policy landscape are explored throughout the semester. For example, when studying house fire deaths among children, the students learned how poverty, substandard housing, and employment policies contribute to the risk of house fires and child injury and mortality. In another semester, when studying rising levels of diabetes, students explored the roles of nutrition, education, and urban-planning policies. When studying student debt, the class examined links among tax, education, and income policies. When studying home foreclosures, students considered the roles of economic, housing, and employment policies. Finally, when studying undocumented immigration, students examined wage, social service, and immigration policies. In other words, while focusing the lens on a particular topic, it was expanded to understand the larger context and how people's experiences "on the ground" are related to public policies.

The policy project also teaches research skills for evidence-based policy practice (Schorr, 2012; Social Work Policy Institute, 2010). Students learn to narrow a policy topic after the first fact-finding assignment. For example, after the class conducted their fact-finding assignment on U. S. immigration, students began to understand why it is important to focus on a specific policy level (federal or state/local), particular age group (children, youth, parents of young children, older adults), geographic location, sexual identity group, or policy area (health, disability, housing, social assistance, nutrition). This process of narrowing a topic requires students to engage with the topic and make key policy practice decisions based on what they had learned. The narrower topic becomes a feasible focus for the remaining assignments.

Policy research also offers opportunities for students to pursue the topic in other courses, in practicums, in their jobs, in their civic lives. They can present and publish results. Each semester we nominate some of the most interesting and promising projects to larger audiences. For instance, we have nominated students for the Influencing State Policy student competitions (http://www.statepolicy.org/), for the university's Undergraduate Research Symposium, and annual Undergraduate Day at the State Capitol (URDC).

In URDC, students create a research poster based on their policy project. The posters are critiqued by faculty and students in preparation for the day when they display their posters—along with those of other students from the other three campuses in the University of Missouri System—in the impressive Rotunda of the Missouri State Capitol. Social work students' posters elicit considerable interest among legislators, aides, and visitors because they often address issues under consideration by state government and elected officials. For example, in 2006, the chairperson of a House Labor Committee, who was sponsoring an increase in the minimum wage, invited the student team to present their findings on "The Effects of Problem Debt on Low-Income Families" at a committee hearing. Their presentation was covered in the university newspaper, *The Current*. Ultimately, the students' testimony aided in the passage of the minimum wage increase. One of the students wrote of the experience:

> We were very fortunate in that we spoke last, and were able to dovetail others' testimony and share data that either supported or refuted earlier testimony. I would not have missed this opportunity. Even before graduation, we were able to raise our voices to address issues that are important to so many of our future clients and fellow human beings.

METHODS AND OUTCOMES

The policy course examined in this article takes place in the bachelor's in social work degree in a mid-size urban land grant university. The course is the second of two required policy courses at the undergraduate level. The first surveys social welfare services with a focus on case management, and the second covers policy development and practice.

The student body is predominately female (87%), a proportion that is similar to other social work programs nationally (CSWE, 2012). However, students in this course are more likely to be minority (46%) (mostly African American) compared to social work students nationally (24% of full time and 30% of part-time students are African American) (CSWE, 2012). Over a third (35%) of students are over age 35, nearly double the national average (18%) (CSWE, 2012). Most of the students in the class have jobs, many full-time. This is reflected in the high proportion of part-time students (44%), compared to the national average (12%) (CSWE, 2012).

Data

Since 2005, we have conducted pre-post surveys of students enrolled in the course, called "Social Issues and Social Policy Development." This section details the methodology and findings. The survey—distinct from the standard course evaluation—is anonymous and approved by the university's Institutional Review Board (IRB). Survey questions include how undergraduate social work students view social policy and their perceptions of learning. The pre- and post-tests were designed to reveal if students developed a better understanding of the specific policy topic, social policy in general, and policy practice by the end of the semester.

Pre-post surveys were administered in 2005, 2006, 2007, 2010, 2011, 2012, and 2013. (Unfortunately, surveys collected in 2008 and 2009 are missing due to loss of data during a move to a different building.) Each class section enrolled 20 to 28 students. Slightly more students completed the pre-tests because some students dropped the class during the semester and did not complete the post-tests.

Survey Instrument

Closed-ended questions. The short survey includes 14 statements, asking students to respond on a 4-point scale (1 = strongly disagree, 2-disagree, 3-agree, 4- strongly agree)[2] about how much they disagree or agree with each statement. Among these statements, six are about the specific topic that semester. For example, in the semester when the class studied household debt and bankruptcy, one of the six statements reads, "I have a good understanding of the range of issues affecting people with household financial problems." The other eight questions address the role of social policy in social work more broadly. For example, one statement reads, "Understanding social policies is important for social workers." Some of these statements ask about students' perceived knowledge/competency related to policy. For example, one reads, "I have experience and knowledge about social policies."

Open-ended questions. In 2010, we added an open-ended question in both the pre-and post-tests: "With all honesty, please describe how you might use what you've learned about [topic] in your work as a social worker."[3] In 2012, we changed this question to: "In your words, describe the role you think social policy plays in social work and the social work profession." We also added a question aimed at eliciting comments on the role of the policy project in student learning by asking them to explain their answer to this question: "Did the policy project help you understand the importance of policy in social work" (possible responses were: It didn't help at all; It helped somewhat; It helped a lot).

Data Analysis

Quantitative data were analyzed mainly by comparing the means in the pre- and post-tests. We identify patterns in the pre- and post-tests. Unfortunately,

---

[2] We intentionally omitted the neutral option on the scale to force students give their opinion. However, "Don't know" is offered as a response category.

[3] Previously, we did not ask for comments because we thought it would take too much time since students also complete a course evaluation for the university. The university course evaluation is now handled online, which allows us to ask students to spend more time on the survey.

significance tests such as paired-samples t-test cannot be used in this analysis because the survey was anonymous and we could not link students' pre-tests and post-tests. A descriptive table is located in Appendix A.

Qualitative data were analyzed using content analysis of open-ended items on the class survey, and on course evaluations. Approximately 75% of the students made an open-ended comment on the survey. Following, we discuss the main themes that emerged from analysis and provide examples, and, where appropriate, provide frequency of certain types of comments.

Quantitative Results

Overall, upon completion of the class, survey results find that students are in more agreement with statements on the survey that address their perceptions of learning. Students reported that the class increased their understanding of social policies and how social policies affect social work in policy formation, how social work practice is affected by social policy, the importance of social policy, and confidence in using a macro approach to helping clients.

Policy formation. One area that shows students' increasing confidence is their understanding of the formation of social policy. For example, more students report they have a good understanding about how bills become laws and how state and federal laws and policies affect social work clients. Figures 1B and 2B in Appendix B show that before taking the policy class, the average level of agreement is below 3 ("agree" on the scale) as compared to mostly above 3 in the post-tests across the observation years, regardless of the specific policy topic selected that semester.

Social work practice and social policy. To find out the extent to which students believe that social policies will affect social work, three questions were asked: (1) I believe social policies will affect my social work career; (2) I understand how social policies will affect my social work practice; and (3) I understand social policies affect social work clients. A visual inspection of the mean scores from pre- and post-tests shows that results for the first question are mixed, but for the other two the results all point to a greater belief among students that social policy can affect their practice and clients (see Appendix A). Most of these increases fall in the range of 0.4–1.0 on the 4-point Likert scale.

Importance of social policy. Students' view of the importance of policy was examined by four items: (1) understanding the importance of social policies for social workers; (2) understanding how to change social policies is important for social workers; (3) understanding the importance of how policies affect people with [specific problems depending on the policy topic]; and (4) understanding the importance of policies and services to help families with [specific problems depending on the policy topic]. The results are quite mixed. Students' consensus to the importance of social policy in social work increased in some semesters but not in other semesters (see Appendix

A). Decreases are even observed in several semesters. A closer look reveals that average ratings for these items are already high in the pre-tests (they all fall between "agree" and "strongly agree"), with some very close to "strongly agree." Our interpretation is that prerequisite courses have already primed undergraduate students to understand that social policy is important in social work practice. As a result, there is not much room left for the policy class to demonstrate improvement in this area. Mixed results may also have to do with the specific student group because within class sections, we found consistency in the results on all four items. For example, in fall 2011 the post-test ratings for the evening class are on average higher than those in the pre-tests, which is completely opposite of the day class (taught by the same instructor) during the same semester.

Confidence in using a macro approach to helping clients. One of the important goals of this class is that students gain knowledge about social policy in general by working on a specific policy topic. This goal is met because at the end of the course more students agree that they have experience and knowledge about social policies (last row of Appendix A). In addition, more students show confidence in understanding and helping clients and their families with a particular problem (depending on the policy topic). Despite some ambiguity, the results are mostly consistent showing the policy class with a specific policy topic may make a difference in students' views about policies related to a particular group. As social workers are expected to work with diverse clients with problems at all levels, such exposure provides students with an example about how to address a problem using a macro approach.

Qualitative Results

Quantitative results do not tell us whether the policy project was helpful. However, open-ended questions provide further insight into quantitative findings. Students' comments suggest that these outcomes are due at least in part to the policy project.

Students' comments focused on three topics: (1) the role of policy in social work, (2) the topic selected for the policy project, and (3) a policy practice perspective.[4] It should be noted that students made more specific observations beginning in 2012 when we added the new question about the value of the policy project in understanding the role of policy in social work practice. In 2012 and 2013, most students said the project helped "a lot" (77%) or "somewhat" (18%), while two said "not at all" (2%) or didn't answer (3%).[5]

---

[4] In the direct quotes, we have made minor corrections in grammar and spelling, such as substituting "effect" for "affect", and "know" for "now". We made no corrections that change the meaning.

[5] One student circled both "a lot" and "somewhat" and was omitted.

Role of policy in social work. Some students commented on how little they knew about policy prior to taking the class: One student observed, *"Basically, I was totally ignorant of any policies before the course"* (2012). Similarly, another wrote: *"I feel like I learned a lot about policy, when I started the course I knew nothing"* (FS 2013).

Several students made some enthusiastic, but rather vague, declarations about policy's significance, such as: *"Social policies make or break what social workers do"* (2010); *"Policies shape what social workers are able to do"* (2010); *"I think social policy almost defines social work, in a way"* (2010). *"Social policy has everything to do with social work"* (2010). *"Social policy affects all aspects of social work in order to help our clients we need social policy and laws to protect, advocate and provide support for them"* (2010).

However, most students' comments were more focused on the role of policy in social work practice. For example, one student wrote that policy *"sets the stage for what we can do or what we should do to help our clients"* (2010). *"The policy project allowed me to see how policies in America affect how and what affects my future clients"* (2012). Some observed they could better *"help clients understand their rights to services"* (2010). Another pointed out: *"I'm more aware of how policy provides and doesn't provide services, especially for Missouri"* (2013). Policy, according to another student, *"plays a Huge role. It will affect all clients and also we need to be aware so we know how and where advocacy is needed"* (2012).

Many comments pointed to the role of policy in providing a statutory and regulatory framework and resources to help clients. One wrote, *"Social policy . . . provides a framework to work within"* (2012), and another pointed out that *"policy affects the way in which social workers practice such as regulations and restrictions on what can be done in practice with clients"* (2012). *"Social policy sets limits (legal and financial) on what social workers can do to help their clients they serve"* (2010). Another learned *"the rules"* by which resources are allocated. *"Being aware of policy gives [social] workers a good idea of how society and laws view and provide for individuals"* (2012). Another pointed out, *"I was able to see there is a lot put into developing policies as a social worker. I must stay on top of changes, needs and resolution to provide quality services"* (2012). Offering a broader perspective, one student said that policy reflects societal values: *"Social policy also dictates what society views as right or wrong"* (2010).

Several students also linked policy to the availability of social work jobs (*"Social policies create our jobs,"* wrote one). Another wrote, *"social policies today will play a role in my career endeavors"* (2010). Another noted that policy could even affect a social worker directly: *"the truth is, many of us are just a paycheck away from being homeless or destitute"* (2012).

The policy topic. Students also reported that they learned about the specific policy topic.[6] A student who was studying immigration policy commented, *"I had no prior understanding of the barriers immigrants faced. I feel it really opened my eyes to things I take for granted"* (2012). Another wrote, *"The seriousness of this problem [home foreclosures] never seemed relevant to my own life until this class"* (2010). Another reflected, *"I had no idea of the importance of this issue [child care] before this class"* (2013), while another wrote about early childhood care, *"It's an issue that I was aware of, but delving into the issues currently surrounding the policy was most helpful"* (2013).

The second type of comment referred to how the new knowledge could help their clients. For instance, after studying household debt, a student gave examples of how to help clients access housing resources: *"I can help them find resources to prevent them from foreclosure, find financial counseling, loan modification, [and] safe refinancing opportunities"* (2010). Another student wrote, *"I think I'll use what I've learned about foreclosure to advocate for education in financial planning and regulation of industries"* (2010). Another student pointed out that, *"Many people I will work with as a social worker may be having housing difficulties because of foreclosures. As I have learned, it not only affects the ones who own the property but also people renting"* (2010). Another student explained how the policy project might be applied in practice: *[A social worker] should know policy because in the future they should be able to advocate on the behalf of homeless bills . . . social workers all should at some point and time advocate for legislation"* (2010).

Adopting a policy practice perspective. The third major area of comments concerned social workers' role in policy change. As one student wrote, *"I'm starting to realize policy is social work and social work is policy. As social workers we need to know and stay up on policy and learn how to advocate for change for policies to help reach out clients in need"* (2013). *"This class really made us realize what it takes to put a policy in action"* (2013). Another student made the connection between studying social policy and knowing what changes are needed: *"We have to understand policy to understand how to lobby and what to lobby for"* (2010). Another asserted, *"In order for social workers to be beneficial in the lives of their clients, they need to be involved in the processes that create policy"* (2011). *"One role of a social worker is being an advocate and social policy is all about advocating for clients and the problems they face"* (2010). Another noted, *"Without the advocacy to ensure changes and continued funding, it will be harder to meet the needs of clients"* (2010).

Some pointed out that this involves learning policy practice skills. Advocacy skills were mentioned by several students, such as these: *"I also

---

[6] This section includes only a few examples of how students might apply knowledge gained from the policy project. There were too many comments to include in this article.

learned how to do some advocacy work" (2010), and "*I will also use the advocacy skills and resources provided to me throughout the rest of my education and possible career*" (2010). Some learned how conceptualize the process of policy practice, "*Prior to this class I didn't have a clue of how to go from start to finish on how to create a change [in] public policy*" (2012), and "*it helped to know how the process works and how I can change a policy and the steps I need to take to make changes to help my clients*" (2012). The policy project in several comments helped students know how to identify gaps and engage in policy change, such as this student who wrote, "*helped me know how policies get changed or enacted to so that when I feel strongly about an issue, I will have a better understanding of how to try to change it*" (2013). Some specifically mentioned research and analysis, such as this student: "*This was helpful to learn what policies need to be changed. The fact that I had researched a ton of information helped*" (2013), and another who noted, "*I learned new methods of gaining information*" (2010).

Some students articulated a growing understanding that social issues are often more complex than at first glance. One student wrote, "*I learned a lot about how one issue is really multiple issues . . . and this will be true when working with families. I had to research multiple things to understand the entire issue and I think this is important*" (2010). Similarly, another student observed: "*It made me really think about every aspect of an issue and how policy affects us*" (2012). For another student, the exercise demonstrated, "*how much work it takes to change a law*" (2012). "*This class really made us realize what it takes to put a policy in action. It also showed us how many ways our clients can be affected by policy*" (2013).

Pedagogy. Finally, although we did not ask specifically about pedagogy, several students made relevant observations. Students commented about doing a policy project and how it helped them learn. One student wrote: "*The research done this semester has helped me to see a Bigger Picture*" (2013). Another student's comment helps to explain that it might be easier to grasp the role of policy when studying one topic in depth: "*I liked that we looked at the policies surrounding one topic. I would have been overwhelmed if we had not focused. . . . [This project] really made us realize what it takes to put a policy in action*" (2012).

Students commented on the way the project was divided "*into pieces*" (2013). "*I like how we started off simple with the fact sheet and built upon the last [policy brief]*" (2012). A strength of the course, according to another student, was "*the different parts that lead up to the policy brief*" (2013).

In contrast, some students commented that the policy project approach was challenging, and they had trouble grasping the purpose of the assignments. The course, in the opinion of one student, "*Definitely pushed you beyond your comfort zone in understanding, examining, and taking action from a social workers' perspective*" (2013). Another student found "*The expectations of the proposal assignment . . . difficult to grasp*" (2013), and another wrote that *"The assignments seemed a little ambiguous and I vaguely understood at times"* (2013).

Other comments regarded the in-depth focus on one topic. Most said it helped their understanding, such as one who wrote, *"In examining one area, it allowed a better understanding of how policy works"* (2013). However, a few students did not like the focus on one topic. One student explained that *"it helped 'a lot' to be able to follow one topic and really see it from all angles, [but] at the same time, I would have liked to explore other topics"* (2012). One student checked "not helpful" and wrote: *"I felt like it was the same info over and over"* (2012).

A few also commented that they would have preferred to pick their own topic, as this student pointed out: *"I felt like allowing us to choose our subject rather than providing one topic for the class reduced interest and personal investment in learning about policy"* (2013). Another student in the class that studied early child care and education wrote: *"I would have gotten a lot more out of this course if we could have picked our topic. Not having children myself, I am not educated nor passionate about childcare issues, and so it would have been more beneficial to choose a topic"* (2013).

Study Limitations

There are limitations to the above findings. Regarding the pre-posttest, although the anonymous class survey encourages participation and honest responses, it does not allow pre-post comparisons using significance tests. Second, we cannot know from this analysis the independent effects of each course component (e.g., policy project, text, instructor, or other factors). Sorting out effects would require more sophisticated research design, which is challenging for many reasons, but particularly because of the difficulty in controlling for differences in instructor style. Third, there could be social desirability bias as the study examines student perceptions of learning. Finally, qualitative evidence (comments from open-ended questions) does not reflect the opinions of all respondents since approximately one-quarter did not write comments.

DISCUSSION AND IMPLICATIONS

This article examines a pedagogical approach to helping often-reluctant undergraduate students make the connection between social policy and people's well-being and life chances, and learn how to incorporate social policy practice into their set of professional skills. Overall, we find that the approach using semester-long topics captured students' attention and made clear the importance of social policy. The strongest quantitative and qualitative evidence suggests that students increase understanding of policy formation and how policies can help people, especially regarding the specific issue studied throughout the semester. This may be important because it coincides with students' motivation to help people.

Comparing different class sections, the pre-post survey evidence is mixed regarding changes in perceptions of the importance of social policy. In part, this is due to relatively high scores in the pre-test. It is possible that at the beginning of the semester students have a vague and general impression that social policy is important, but gain a more tangible understanding of what this means and how social policy affects social work practice. Qualitative evidence suggests students developed greater depth of understanding about the importance of policy.

Quantitative results concerning the role of policy in students' careers are similarly mixed. Students reported that policy would affect their practice, but their responses suggest that it would not affect their careers. These findings deserve more research attention. It could be that while students do not envision policy practice as a career, they do gain understanding about how policy affects clients and social work practice. It also could mean they have not fully absorbed the nature of the link between policy and social work.

Qualitative comments suggest that the four-part policy project increasingly drew students in. However, the qualitative evidence also raises some pedagogical challenges. The decision to focus on one topic suggests a trade-off between what may be beneficial to a majority of students compared to a few who wish to pursue a topic of their own. At the undergraduate foundation level, the benefits of focusing on one topic may outweigh the disadvantages. For example, there is a benefit to bringing in a series of speakers who offer a range of perspectives on a single topic. Focusing class discussions on policy areas through the lens of a particular topic, and generating collective knowledge about a topic led to more sophisticated policy discussions by the end of the semester. At the graduate level, however, students often are more focused on a particular area of practice, and therefore this approach may not work as well.

This study increases knowledge about a promising approach to teaching policy practice with research evidence of successes over seven semesters. The evaluation built in the new teaching practice allows the educators to know precisely the outcomes of this approach. As social work educators are increasingly and creatively using experiential learning in teaching policy practice, such evaluations are not only important but also essential to informing discussions on a larger scale. Future research should consider a comparison group that is taught in a more traditional way. However, to control for instructor quality, it would be ideal if the treatment group and the comparison group both are taught by the same instructor. It would also be helpful to use a survey instrument that measures not only students' perceptions of learning but also objective measures of knowledge and skills in policy practice. Finally, the class survey questionnaire may be revised by adding identifiers and some questions about student characteristics (such as indicators of traditional vs. nontraditional student). This will not only allow significance tests and estimation of the effect size but also allow researchers to know how survey results may differ by student characteristics. Finally, research that assesses the long-term effects of instructional approaches on students' future course and career decisions would also be helpful.

CONCLUSION

A key challenge in teaching social policy is how to help social work students grasp the "bigger picture" and understand that there are many ways to help many people, including through policy change. Studying one policy topic in depth is a promising approach to pedagogy that may improve student learning, as well as help students envision policy practice roles. This article suggests that this kind of experiential approach may spark interest and address attitudes and motivation to engage in policy practice. Using mixed methods, the evidence suggests that the policy project makes policy come alive and gives students a way to visualize a professional role in social policy practice. For many students, perhaps most, this is a different role than they imagined assuming as a professional social worker.

ACKNOWLEDGMENTS

An early version of this article was presented at the Research on Policy Practice Symposium, The Institute for Advanced Studies, The Hebrew University of Jerusalem, January 28, 2013. The authors wish to thank the many undergraduate students enrolled in our social policy courses over the years who contributed to this article through their participation and reactions to the curriculum.

REFERENCES

Abell, N., & McDonell, J. R. (1990). Preparing for practice: Motivations, expectations and aspirations of the MSW class of 1990. *Journal of Social Work Education*, *26*, 57–64.

Abramovitz, M. (1993). Should all social work students be educated for social change? *Journal of Social Work Education*, *29*(1), 6–11.

American Academy of Social Work and Social Welfare. (2013, November). *Grand accomplishments in social work* (Grand Challenges for Social Work Initiative, Working Paper No. 2). Baltimore, MD: Author.

Anderson, D. K., & Harris, B. M. (2005). Teaching social welfare policy: A comparison of two pedagogical approaches. *Journal of Social Work Education, 41*(3), 511–526.

Bogo, M., Raphael, D., Roberts, R. (1993). Interests, activities, and self-identification among social work students: Toward a definition of social work identity. *Journal of Social Work Education, 29*(3), 1043–1097.

Butler, A. C. (1990). A reevaluation of social work students' career interests. *Journal of Social Work Education, 26*, 45–56.

Butler, A. C. (1992). The attractions of private practice. *Journal of Social Work Education, 28*, 47–60.

Chandler, M. A. (2013, April 29). State funding for preschool drops as Obama calls for expansion. *The Washington Post*. Retrieved from http://www.washingtonpost.com/local/education/state-funding-for-preschool-drops-as-obama-calls-for-expansion/2013/04/28/70778f5a-afae-11e2-a986-eec837b1888b_story.html

Christie, L. (2008, January 29). Foreclosures up 75% in 2007. CNN Money. Retrieved from http://money.cnn.com/2008/01/29/real_estate/foreclosure_filings_2007/

Clark, E. J. (2007). From the director: Advocacy: Profession's cornerstone, July. Washington DC: NASW.

Council on Social Work Education. (2008). Educational Policy and Accreditation Standards. Alexandria, VA: CSWE. Retrieved from http://www.cswe.org/Accreditation/2008EPASDescription.aspx

Council on Social Work Education (2012). 2012 Annual Statistics on Social Work Education in the United States. Washington, DC: CSWE. Retrieved from http://www.cswe.org/File.aspx?id=68989

Cummins, L. K., Byers, K. V., & Pedrick, L. (2011, updated). *Policy Practice for Social Workers: New Strategies for a New Era*. New York, NY: Pearson.

Dewey, J. (1938). *Experience in education*. Retrieved from http://www.ruby.fgcu.edu

Dochy, F., Segers, M., Van Den Bossche, P., & Gijbels, D. (2003). Effects of problem-based learning: A meta-analysis. 533-568. *Learning and Instruction, 13*, 533–568.

Figueira-McDonough, J. (1993). Policy practice: The neglected side of social work intervention. *Social Work, 38*(2), 179–188.

Fisher, R., & Corciullo, D. (2011). Rebuilding community organizing education in social work. *Journal of Community Practice, 19*(4), 355–368.

Freeman, E. M. (1996). Welfare reforms and services for children and families: Setting a new practice, research, and policy agenda. *Social Work, 41*(5), 521–532.

Gibbons, J., & Gray, M. (2002). An integrated and experience-based approach to social work education: The Newcastle model. *Social Work Education, 21*, 529–549.

Gibbons, J., & Gray, M. (2005). Teaching social work students about social policy. *Australian Social Work, 58*(1), 58–75.

Glater, J. D. (2008, October 17). In a downturn, college strains family budgets. *New York Times*. Retrieved from http://www.nytimes.com/2008/10/17/business/17student.html?pagewanted=all&_r=0

Hmelo-Silver, C. E. (2004). Problem-based learning: What and how do students learn? *Educational Psychology Review, 16*, 235–266.

Hoefer, R. (2006). *Advocacy practice for social justice*. Chicago, IL: Lyceum.

Hymans, D. (2000). Teaching BSW students community practice using an interdisciplinary neighborhood needs assessment project. *Journal of Baccalaureate Social Work, 5*(2), 81–92.

Iatridis, D. S. (1995). Policy practice. In R. L. Edwards (Ed.), *Encyclopedia of social work* (19th ed.) (pp. 1855–1866). Washington, DC: NASW Press.

Jansson, B. S. (2010). Becoming an effective policy advocate (6th edition). Pacific Grove, CA: Brooks/Cole.

Jansson, B. S., Fertig, R., Hansung, K., & Heidemann, G. (2011). Practicing policy, pursuing change, and promoting social justice: A policy instructional approach. *Journal of Social Work Education, 47*(1), 37–52

Johnson, A. K. (2004). Social work is standing on the legacy of Jane Addams, but are we sitting on the sidelines? *Social Work, 49*(2), 319–322.

Kleinfield, N. R. (2006, January 9). Diabetes and its awful toll quietly emerge as a crisis. *New York Times*. Retrieved from http://www.nytimes.com/2006/01/09/nyregion/nyregionspecial5/09diabetes.html?pagewanted=all&_r=0

Klinenberg, E. (2002). *Heat wave: A social autopsy of disaster in Chicago*. Chicago, IL: University of Chicago Press.

Kolb, A., & Kolb, D. A. (2008). Experiential learning theory: A dynamic, holistic approach to management learning, education and development. In S. Armstrong, & C. Fukami (Eds.), *The SAGE handbook of management learning, education and development* (pp. 42–69). London, England: Sage. doi:10.4135/9780857021038.n3

Linhorst, D. M. (2002). Federalism and social justice: Implications for social work. *Social Work, 47*(3), 201–208.

NASW. (2008). Code of ethics of the National Association of Social Workers. Washington, DC: NASW. Retrieved from http://www.socialworkers.org

NASW. (2011). *Social work dictionary* (5th ed.). Washington, DC: NASW Press.

Nuckles, C. R. (2000). Student-centered teaching: Making it work. *Adult Learning, 11*, 5–7.

Pew Research Center (2013, October 18). Trust in government nears record low, but most federal agencies are viewed favorably. Pew Research Center for People and the Press. Retrieved from http://www.people-press.org/2013/10/18/trust-in-government-nears-record-low-but-most-federal-agencies-are-viewed-favorably/

Rocha, C. J. (2000). Evaluating experiential teaching methods in a policy practice course: The case for service learning to increase political participation. *Journal of Social Work Education, 36*, 53–63.

Rocha, C. J. (2007). *Essentials of social policy practice*. Hoboken, NJ: John Wiley & Sons.

Rocha, C. J., & Johnson, A. K. (1997). Teaching family policy through a policy practice framework. *Journal of Social Work Education, 33*, 433–444.

Rothman, J. (2012, October). Education for macro intervention a survey of problems and prospects (Issue brief). Lynwood, IL: Association for Community Organization and Social Administration.

Rothman, J., & Mizrahi, T. (2014). *Balancing micro and macro practice: A challenge for social work. Social Work, 59*(1), 91–93. doi:10.1093/sw/swt067

Rubin, A., & Johnson, P. J. (1984). Direct practice interests of entering MSW students. *Journal of Education for Social Work, 20*(2), 5–16.

Rubin, A., Johnson, P. J., & DeWeaver, K. L. (1986). Direct practice interests of MSW students: Changes from entry to graduation. *Journal of Social Work Education, 22*(2), 98–108.

Schorr, L. B. (2012). Broader evidence for bigger impact. *Stanford Social Innovation Review.* Retrieved from http://www.lisbethschorr.org/doc/Fall_2012_Broader_Evidence_for_Bigger_Impact.pdf

Semple, K. (2011, May 21). Illegal Immigrants' Underground Lives Hobble Their U.S.-Born Children, Study Says. *New York Times,* A17. Retrieved from http://www.nytimes.com/2011/05/21/nyregion/illegal-immigrants-children-suffer-study-finds.html

Sewpaul, V., & Jones, D. (2004). Global Standards for Social Work Education and Training. International Association of Schools of Social Work and the International Federation of Social Workers, adopted at the General Assemblies of IASSW and IFSW, Adelaide, Australia. Retrieved from http://cdn.ifsw.org/assets/ifsw_65044-3.pdf

Sherraden, M. S., Slosar, B., & Sherraden, M. (2002). Innovation in social policy: Researcher, practitioner, advocate, and student collaboration. *Social Work, 47*(3), 209–224.

Social Work Policy Institute. (2012). Influencing social policy: Positioning social work graduates for policy careers. Critical conversation brief. Washington, DC: NASW. Retrieved from http://www.acosa.org/joomla/pdf/InfluencingSocialPolicyBrief.pdf

Specht, H., & Courtney, M. (1994). *Unfaithful angels: How social work has abandoned its mission.* New York, NY: The Free Press.

Sternberg, S. (2011, February 16). Report: Half of children killed in fires are under age 5. *USA Today.* Retrieved from http://usatoday30.usatoday.com/news/nation/2011-02-14-kidsinfire14_ST_N.htm

Walz, T., & Groze, V. (1991). The mission of social work revisited: An agenda for 1990s. *Social Work, 36*(6), 500–504.

Weiss, I., Gal, J., Cnaan, R. A., & Maglajlic, R. (2002). What kind of social policy do social work students prefer? A comparison of students in three countries. *International Social Work, 45*(1), 59–81.

Weiss, I., Gal, J., & Dixon, J. (Eds.). (2003). *Professional ideologies and preferences in social work: A global study.* Westport, CT: Praeger.

Weiss, I., Gal, J., & Katan, J. (2006). Social policy for social work: A teaching agenda. *British Journal of Social Work, 36,* 789–806.

Weiss-Gal, I., & Savaya, R. (2012). Teaching policy practice: A hands-on seminar for social workers in Israel. *Journal of Policy Practice, 11*(3), 139–157.

Whitaker, T., & Arrington, P. (2008). Social worker at work. NASW Membership Workforce Study. Washington, DC: National Association of Social Workers. Retrieved from http://workforce.socialworkers.org/studies/SWatWork.pdf

Wolk, J. L., Pray, J. E., Weismiller, T., & Dempsey, D. (1996). Political practica: Educating social work students for policymaking. *Journal of Social Work Education, 32*(1), 91–100.

Wyers, N. L. (1990). Policy practice in social work: Models and issues. *Journal of Social Work Education, 27*(3), 241–251.

Zull, J. E. (2004). The art of changing the brain. *Teaching for Meaning, 62*(1), 68–72.

APPENDIX A

TABLE A1 Descriptive Results from the Pre- and Posttests [a]

Questions	Fall 2005* evening (n = 22)		Fall 2006** (n = 19)		Fall 2007** (n = 20)		Fall 2010* (day) (n = 20)		Fall 2010* (evening) (n = 20)		Fall 2011*** (Day) (n = 23)		Fall 2011*** (evening) (n = 22)		Fall 2012*** (day) (n = 23)		Fall 2012*** (evening) (n = 23)		Fall 2013**** (day) (n = 28)		Fall 2013**** (evening) (n = 27)	
	Pre	Post	Pre	Post	Pre	Post	Pre	Post	Pre	Post	Pre	Post	Pre	Post	Pre	Post	Pre	Post	Pre	Post	Pre	Post
Social work practice and social policy																						
I believe social policies will affect my social work career	3.60	3.87	3.72	3.94	3.74	3.50	3.68	3.71	3.63	3.44	3.68	3.63	3.86	3.93	3.86	3.63	3.94	4.00	4.14	4.08	3.70	3.82
I understand how social policies will affect my social work practice	2.65	3.67	2.88	3.63	3.00	3.33	3.19	3.50	2.84	3.41	2.91	3.35	3.05	3.67	3.00	3.57	3.50	3.86	3.21	3.84	3.07	3.55
I understand how social policies affect social work clients	2.86	3.80	3.13	3.69	3.25	3.50	3.30	3.74	2.85	3.47	3.00	3.29	3.23	3.69	3.00	3.52	3.39	3.79	3.14	3.88	3.27	3.68
Importance of social policy																						
Understanding social policies is important for the social work profession in general	3.65	3.93	3.63	3.82	3.89	3.38	3.83	4.00	3.85	3.47	3.86	3.77	3.73	4.00	3.81	3.70	3.78	4.00	4.04	4.12	3.93	3.95
Understanding how to change social policies is important for social workers	3.45	3.73	3.68	3.76	3.78	3.50	3.57	3.77	3.56	3.53	3.78	3.56	3.64	3.87	3.85	3.62	3.61	3.92	3.82	4.12	3.74	3.77
It is important for social workers to understand how policies affect people with . . .	3.63	3.73	3.53	3.94	3.68	3.50	3.79	3.88	3.74	3.69	3.77	3.56	3.77	3.87	3.85	3.70	3.67	3.92	3.89	4.08	3.78	3.68
It is important for social workers to understand about policies and services to help families with . . .	3.57	3.73	3.56	3.94	3.79	3.50	3.75	3.88	3.84	3.75	3.77	3.63	3.73	3.80	3.85	3.68	3.72	4.00	3.93	4.04	3.89	3.73

As a social worker, I expect to assist clients who....	3.43	3.44	3.24	3.59	3.59	3.38	3.75	3.71	3.35	3.47	3.70	3.50	3.41	3.63	3.53	3.52	3.69	3.65	3.14	3.72	3.54	3.41
I have a good understanding of the range of issues affecting people with ...	2.55	3.00	2.74	3.65	3.00	3.33	3.00	3.47	2.89	3.20	2.21	3.29	2.38	3.57	2.75	3.32	2.83	3.57	2.79	3.68	3.30	3.36
I have a good understanding about how policies and services can help people prevent ...	2.64	3.00	2.42	3.65	2.44	3.11	2.81	3.42	2.50	3.13	2.14	3.24	2.19	3.50	2.25	3.29	2.72	3.64	2.61	3.68	3.11	3.36
I have a good understand about how to help families with a member who has ...	2.20	3.12	2.32	3.47	2.32	3.33	2.74	3.32	2.47	3.19	2.14	3.19	2.10	3.31	2.25	3.36	2.72	3.60	2.93	3.68	3.07	3.41
I have experience and knowledge about social policies	2.45	3.44	2.35	3.59	2.80	3.22	2.74	3.11	2.50	3.19	2.45	2.88	2.59	3.13	2.36	3.23	2.94	3.46	2.50	3.24	2.70	3.14

*Policy project focuses on family problem debt.
***Policy project focuses on diabetes.*
****Policy project focuses on immigrants and refugees.*
*****Policy project focuses on early childhood care.*
Grey areas indicate that the post-test mean is higher than the pre-test mean.

APPENDIX B

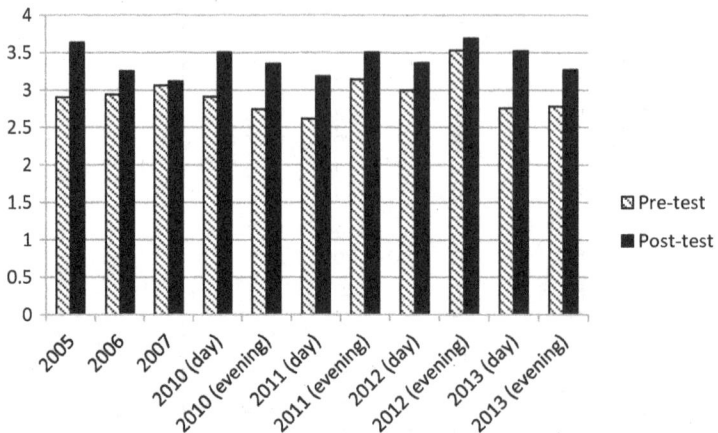

FIGURE B1 "I have a good understanding about how bills become laws."

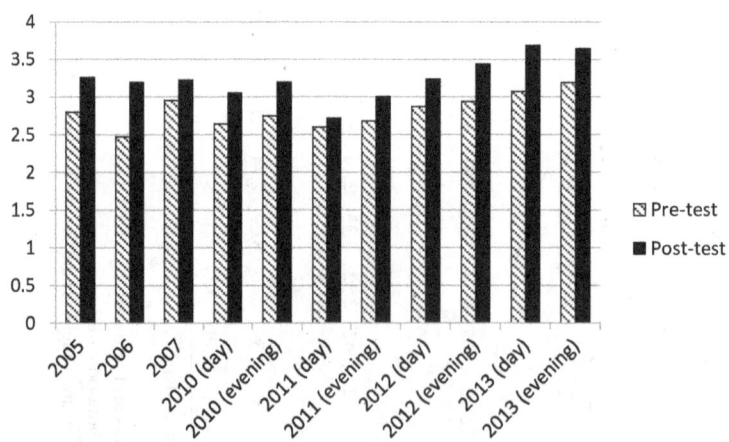

FIGURE B2 "I have a good understanding about how state and federal laws and policies affect social work clients."

Embracing Applied Policy Practice: A Case Study From a Robust BSW Program

ELIZABETH TWINING BLUE and LYNN AMERMAN GOERDT
Social Work, University of Wisconsin–Superior, Superior, Wisconsin, USA

This article, first presented at the Policy Conference 2.0 in Austin, Texas, May 2014, portrays a case example of an undergraduate social work program's robust response to the imperative that policy advocacy serve as a demonstration to students of commitment to the profession and its mission. Initial evidence from field supervisors, students, and examples of recognition suggests that students are prepared to engage in policy advocacy as they enter the profession.

INTRODUCTION

Instruction at the undergraduate level offers social work programs a critical opportunity to influence social work students and teach them how to conduct effective policy advocacy. This is especially important because social work practitioners have a professional obligation to use policy advocacy knowledge and skills to bring about social and economic justice for underserved and underrepresented groups. Infusion of policy advocacy within a program's policy sequence serves as a demonstration to its students of its central role in practice. This case example offers a discussion of how one program approached embedding such instruction into its curriculum, particularly within its policy sequence, engaging its students in experiential learning activities.

Social Policy Advocacy Instruction in the United States and Abroad

As countries around the world have witnessed decreasing social protections, global leaders have called on social workers to lead and/or partner in social policy advocacy efforts. In many European countries, austerity measures have begun to erode the social protection measures that have been critical to efforts of social equality (Hammarberg as cited in de Chenu, 2012).

The 2012 Joint World Conference on Social Work and Social Development set the stage for a renewed emphasis on social workers fulfilling the mission of the profession by engaging in policy practice and advocacy. In the opening ceremony of the conference, Holmberg-Herrstrom introduced the Global Agenda for Social Action, a collaborative agenda between three international social work organizations, and outlined a commitment for social workers to engage in advocating for systems that address oppression and inequality (as cited in de Chenu, 2012). Holmberg-Herrstrom (2012) also identified the solidification and expansion of social protection floors as an important aspect of this commitment. Many of the plenary sessions at the conference also focused on the importance of social policy practice and advocacy. However, Gal & Weiss-Gal (2013) have pointed out that this kind of practice and advocacy appears to be lacking in many countries. They have further explained that although many of the social democratic countries have committed to incorporating social policy practice and advocacy into their social work instruction, this has not translated into action.

In the United States, lack of social protections has fueled a demand for social work educators and practitioners to engage in social welfare policy advocacy. Hoefer (2013) stated that the reality is that the United States is the only industrialized country with such a state of affairs. It is ironic that this deplorable condition has led to embedding skills of policy advocacy and practice in the social work curriculum to an extent that appears unprecedented in industrialized countries (Gal & Weiss-Gal, 2013). The expectation for social workers to be engaged in policy practice is communicated in social work education, particularly in the United States, to be a mandatory part of their practice, no matter the setting (Anderson & Harris, 2005; Gal & Weiss-Gal, 2013; Gibbons & Gray, 2005; Heidemann, Fertig, Jansson, & Kim, 2011; Hoefer, 2013; Weiss, Gal, & Katan, 2006). The commitment to social policy practice and advocacy is explicitly and frequently mentioned in the literature, discourse, and codes of ethics (Gal & Weiss-Gal, 2013).

The evidence typically offered as a demonstration of the commitment to social workers as social policy practitioners is analysis of the extent to which accreditation agencies and primary national social work associations are explicit in their accrediting expectations and codes of ethics (Gal & Weiss-Gal, 2013). At the same time, however, there is a disturbing trend that this commitment has not translated into practice (Gal & Weiss-Gal, 2013; Hoefer, 2013).

The reasons for the discrepancy between expectation and actual engagement are numerous. They include:

1. limited inclusion of policy practice courses in the curricula;
2. national individualism ethos;
3. lack of agency-norms for policy practice;
4. limited interest of students; and
5. lack of social work faculty with expertise in policy practice (Gal & Weiss-Gal, 2006, 2013).

Gibbons and Gray (2005) have also declared social policy should not be taught at the periphery of social work education, but rather should be integrated into the curriculum.

Many current efforts move forward to address this. Such efforts may be found at the educational level; in social work education, they are imbedded in the accreditation standards social work programs must meet, in the professional organization codes of ethics being taught, in the renewal and development of inclusive curriculum, and in the fostering of innovative teaching strategies.

Influence of Accrediting Body and Professional Organizations

In the United States, social work education is governed by the Council on Social Work Education (CSWE); its Educational Policy and Accreditation Standards (EPAS) make explicit the expectation for social policy advocacy and practice primarily in two standard areas: 2.1.5, "advancing human rights and social and economic justice"; and 2.1.8, "engage in policy practice to advance social and economic well-being and to deliver effective social work services" (CSWE, 2008). Typically, social work education programs have responded to the standards by incorporating social welfare policy courses at both the bachelors and masters level (Gal &Weiss-Gal, 2013).

The National Association of Social Work Code of Ethics includes language in which it outlines a professional expectation of conducting policy advocacy. The preamble for its Code of Ethics states, "Social workers promote social justice. . . . These activities may be in the form of direct practice, community organizing, supervision, consultation administration, advocacy, social and political action, policy development and implementation, education, and research and evaluation" (NASW, 2008). Specifically, Section 6.04, Social and Political Action, states clearly that social workers are expected to engage in political advocacy and participation as a way to meet their ethical responsibility to the broader society. Hoefer (2013, p. 172) describes NASW as the "focal point for political action" in the United States.

Responses to Increased Need for Teaching Social Welfare Policy Advocacy

To address the need for expanded teaching of social welfare policy advocacy and practice, two primary approaches appear to be utilized most often: integrating policy skills and practice into the broad social work curriculum and expanding course offerings related to policy advocacy and practice.

Gibbons and Gray (2005) argue that social workers are more likely to engage in policy practice in the field if it is integrated throughout all courses. They reject the teaching of policy as "bifurcated" content, and they are particularly critical of the traditional teaching of micro vs macro practice, believing that this tends to limit the extent that social workers view policy advocacy and practice as a necessary component in fulfilling the mission of the profession. Henman (2012) has suggested modifications be made to the teaching pedagogy, specifically adding policy teaching strategies intended to engage student's interests. Strategies suggested included providing clear examples of social workers engaging in social policy practice, introducing a weekly "hot policy topic" at the beginning of each class, and requiring students to observe governmental policymakers in action (p. 345). Rocha (2000) maintains that social work students who participate in experiential learning activities are more likely to engage in post-graduate policy advocacy than those who do not. Practicing advocacy as a student could increase the likelihood of advocacy in the profession, having a significant impact on the extent that social workers are engaged in the practice of policy advocacy. This point of view is echoed by Anderson and Harris (2005); they intentionally incorporated service learning into their teaching and final internship to engage students in experiential pedagogy and have been able to demonstrate success in developing students' policy-related skills.

In order to understand the extent to which regional social work programs have expanded course offerings related to social policy advocacy and practice, the authors reviewed course descriptions on the websites of 39 CSWE accredited BSW programs in four Midwestern states. The review indicated four programs (10%) had two policy courses, with one of these courses clearly incorporating policy advocacy activities. Seventeen programs (44%) alluded to using advocacy activities in one policy course. Sixteen programs (41%) had one policy course, and the programs' course descriptions did not mention policy advocacy or practice at all. Finally, two schools (5%) offered two policy courses, with neither course description explicitly including policy advocacy nor practice activities. It appears numerous programs from this region may not yet have made an overt commitment to promotion and instruction of policy advocacy in their policy curricula. The case study program described below was one of the four programs offering two policy courses and with overt policy advocacy activities included in course descriptions; it also includes its introductory course as a third course in its policy focused curriculum sequence.

UNITED STATES BACCALAUREATE CASE EXAMPLE

The following case example describes a social work program that intentionally expanded social policy advocacy and practice throughout its curriculum, as well as modified its pedagogy to incorporate innovative and engaging teaching strategies. The case example discusses the background of the program, the transition of its focused curriculum (social policy advocacy and practice), and the documented outcomes associated with this transition.

Background of Social Work Program

The program was located on a small public liberal arts university situated in the upper Midwest of the United States, in a community bordering another state. Steady enrollment of social work students occurred over the 10-year timespan in which the shift in social policy teaching occurred. The program had 102 students admitted to the social work program in 2003 (approximately 4% of the 2,527 total students enrolled and in 2012 had 110 students, or just over 4% of the 2,550 total students enrolled). Its students were being prepared primarily for rural and small community social work practice, both in the state in which the university was located as well as the state it bordered.

History of Transition to Three-Course Policy Sequence

Over the course of approximately three years, the social work program transitioned from a two-course policy sequence to a three-course sequence. The transition was driven by student outcome data, discussions with other social work educators, and began in earnest in 2003.

Feedback from student self-efficacy survey data and professional colleagues. The Social Work Program Student Advisory Committee conducts an annual Social Work Outcome Survey of students to receive information on their learning experience and the extent that the curriculum has effectively met student needs. Between 2001 and 2004, results consistently demonstrated that students had relatively low perceptions about their abilities to use policy advocacy knowledge and skills, typically rating themselves as having some to good ability. Table 1 includes the range of mean scores

TABLE 1 Table Representing Extent Senior Students Felt They Mastered Policy Advocacy and Practice Objectives Fully and Mostly (2001–2004), by Range of Mean on 6-point Scale

Policy Advocacy and Practice Course Goal and Objective	4-Year Range of Mean
A. To assess the structure of organizations, service delivery systems and communities	3.7–4.5
B. To apply lessons from the history of social work practice to current practice situations	3.9–4.1
C. To analyze current social welfare policies using a social welfare lens.	3.6–4.4
D. To advocate for change with and on behalf of macro level clients.	3.6–4.5

Note. 6-point scale; 1 = very little ability to 6 = very strong ability; $N = 56$.

for four years of data using a 6-point scale (1 = very little ability to 6 = very strong ability), which are between a 3.6 and 4.5.

The evaluations for the junior level course specifically focused on policy, (Social Welfare Policy and Services), also included comments from students indicating that they did not feel prepared to engage in policy advocacy and practice. For example, in the 2004 course evaluation, one student commented that the course could be improved with "More focus on actual policies & how to go about them". In addition, students had come to their advisors stating that they did not understand the purpose for the course and did not see the value of the policy course in relation to their future social work practice.

This message was consistent with national discussions facilitated by CSWE and Association of Baccalaureate Social Work Program Directors (BPD) in which program faculty were participating. In response to the feedback on policy practice preparation, the faculty began introducing additional policy content into the Introduction to Social Work course and established a plan to significantly expand policy-focused teaching into two courses instead of the previous single course. Beginning in 2005, the program converted the single policy focused course into a two-course sequence; Ecology of Social Welfare Policy Making and Social Welfare Policy Practice This resulted in the current three-course policy sequence.

Curriculum response. The Introduction to Social Work course established the foundation for students to begin to understand the development of the profession in the context of social welfare history and to begin to understand the relationship between social welfare issues and policies. Students learned how contexts are changing and the ways in which social workers are engaged in social change efforts.

The second course in the sequence, Ecology of Social Welfare Policy Making, was designed to focus on the context and background of policy-making. Course goals and objectives were focused on student understanding of social welfare policy within its social, political, historical, cultural, and economic environments. Much effort in course instruction focused on establishing the context of policymaking, particularly the history of social welfare policy in the United States. In the redesigned course, students were engaged in numerous application activities and short-term team projects; they were encouraged from the beginning to find connections to an issue about which they were passionate and the extent to which that issue has been impacted or resolved through social welfare policy.

Examples of assignments in the course included in-depth exploration of social welfare history in the United States as well as a policy analysis assignment. The exploration of social welfare history resulted in the creation of a video on social welfare history in which each student investigates an era in United States history that had a significant impact on social welfare policy development. The eras ranged from pre-Colonial times to more recent events such as the 1969 Stonewall Rebellion in Greenwich Village, New York. The social policy analysis assignment consisted of a policy analysis comparison paper between the United States and a country of the students' choice. Examples of recent comparative topics included violence against women, human trafficking, homelessness, aging-out of foster care, juvenile justice, and mental health care access. For another assignment, the students participated in social work advocacy days at the state capitol. To prepare for this event, students typically investigated current policy issues and prepared themselves to advocate individually or in groups with elected officials.

The third course, Social Welfare Policy Practice, was designed to focus on the student mastery of policy practice skills including advocacy. It was viewed as an additional methods course, focusing on policy practice. An emphasis was on the application of critical thinking skills and the analysis of social welfare policy with the intent to advocate on behalf of or against a policy solution to a social welfare issue.

The formative assignments in this course included a major policy advocacy assignment, engagement in electoral politics, analysis of agency level policy, and an in-depth analysis of topics of oppression and resistance. The policy advocacy activity was a semester long project which begins with the exploration of the student's passions and culminates with the development and presentation of a policy advocacy brief to a publically elected official who has influence on the particular issue. The topics for the policy advocacy briefs are selected by the small teams of students and in the fall of 2013 they included: human trafficking with an emphasis on trafficking of Native American women and girls, needle exchange programs, homelessness, educational inequity and rising cost of textbooks, and connection between animal abuse and domestic violence.

Immediately after the transition, student evaluations began to reflect on the value of the content and activities, connecting it to their future practice. In recent evaluations, when asked about the strengths of the class, students have commented: "Great practical assignments," "The involvement in the community. Policy brief, election assignment," and "Identifying current issues/policies and tackling them."

Imbedding the EPAS competencies. The 2008 EPAS put a renewed emphasis on policy practice, validating the redesign of the policy sequence. The program had traditionally used competency-based course evaluations but to make this more explicit the CSWE (2008) EPAS competencies were formally incorporated into the program's policy courses in 2012, as shown in Table 2, operationalizing the practice behaviors. As mentioned, Introduction to Social Work was integral in introducing policy advocacy concepts into the curriculum, which were further reinforced in Ecology of Social Welfare Policy and then applied in Social Welfare Policy Practice. In examining this table the reader can see how foundation ideas and information on policy and policy advocacy are introduced in the first course; how additional ideas are added in the second course and earlier ideas reinforced there; and finally, how in the third course these are further reinforced and mature concepts and skills relating to policy and policy advocacy are to be mastered by students.

Outcomes of Curriculum Investments

The authors used three data sources to express the extent to which students have achieved the intended outcomes following the shift in curriculum:

1. evidence from program student learning goal outcome data (field supervisor evaluations);
2. evidence from a student self-efficacy measure, *Measuring Achievement of Course Goals, Objectives and Outcomes* conducted at the end of each course; and
3. anecdotal and other evidence of recognition received by students relating to their policy projects.

Evidence from field supervisor evaluations. Prior to the transition to three-course policy sequence, policy practice skills were evaluated by field supervisors as not an area of strength for students, validating the student's own assessment of their skills. After the transition, field supervisors noted a different perception of student's readiness to engage in policy advocacy and practice. Tables 3 and 4 reflect field supervisors' judgment of student competence on objectives related to policy advocacy and practice from 2008 to 2013; Table 3 applys the practice goals and objectives and Table 4 applys the 2008 EPAS competences after they were integrated into the curriculum. All of these students would have experienced the new policy curriculum and teaching strategies. Over the four-year span, there was an increasing trend on all objectives as students were consistently evaluated at or above the expected level for students completing their BSW degree and entering

TABLE 2 How EPAS is Connected to Policy-Focused Course Outcomes

EPAS Statement (2008)	Practice Behaviors incorporated in The Ecology of Social Welfare Policy Making:	Practice Behaviors incorporated in Social Welfare Policy Practice:
Educational Policy 2.1.1 Identify as a professional social worker and conduct oneself accordingly.	A: Advocate for client access to the services of social work B: Practice personal reflection and self-correction to ensure continual professional development C: Attend to professional roles and boundaries	A: Advocate for client access to the services of social work C: Attend to professional roles and boundaries
Educational Policy 2.1.3 Apply critical thinking to inform and communicate professional judgments	C: Tolerate ambiguity in resolving ethical conflicts D: Apply strategies of ethical reasoning to arrive at principled decisions.	D: Apply strategies of ethical reasoning to arrive at principled decisions.
Educational Policy 2.1.4 Engage diversity and difference in practice	A: Distinguish, appraise and integrate multiple sources of knowledge, including research knowledge and practice wisdom B: Analyze models of assessment, prevention, intervention, and evaluation C: Demonstrate effective oral and written communication in working with individuals, families, groups, organizations, communities, and colleagues. A: Recognize the extent to which a culture's structures and values may oppress, marginalize, alienate, or create or enhance power. D: View themselves as learners and engage those with whom they work as informants.	A: Distinguish, appraise and integrate multiple sources of knowledge, including research knowledge and practice wisdom B: Analyze models of assessment, prevention, intervention, and evaluation C: Demonstrate effective oral and written communication in working with individuals, families, groups, organizations, communities, and colleagues. A: Recognize the extent to which a culture's structures and values may oppress, marginalize, alienate, or create or enhance power. D: View themselves as learners and engage those with whom they work as informants.
Education Policy 2.1.5 Advance human rights and social and economic justice		A: Understand the forms and mechanisms of oppression and discrimination B: Advocate for human rights and social and economic justice

(Continued)

TABLE 2 (Continued)

EPAS Statement (2008)	Practice Behaviors incorporated in The Ecology of Social Welfare Policy Making:	Practice Behaviors incorporated in Social Welfare Policy Practice:
Educational Policy 2.1.8 Engage in policy practice to advance social and economic well-being and to deliver effective social work services.	A: Understand the forms and mechanisms of oppression and discrimination B: Advocate for human rights and social and economic justice	B: Collaborate with colleagues and clients for effective policy action.
Educational Policy 2.1.9 Respond to contexts that shape practice	B: Collaborate with colleagues and clients for effective policy action.	A: Continuously discover, appraise, and attend to changing locales, populations, scientific and technological advances, and emerging societal trends to provide relevant services.

TABLE 3 Extent Field Supervisors Judged Students Demonstrated Competence on Policy Advocacy and Practice Objectives (2008–2011), Mean Levels of Agreement on a 4-Point Scale

Policy Advocacy and Practice Course Goal and Objective	2008–2009	2009–2010	2010–2011
4.1 Can appraise the structure of organizations	3.1	3.3	3.3
4.2 Can appraise the structure of service delivery systems	3.1	3.1	3.2
4.3 Can appraise the structure of communities	3.0	3.1	3.2
4.4 Can, under supervision, advocate effectively for organizational change based on the principles of social and economic justice	3.1	3.1	3.2
4.5 Can, under supervision, advocate effectively for community change based on the principles of social and economic justice	3.1	3.2	3.2
5.1 Can integrate knowledge of the history of social work profession with the ability to analyze its impact upon client systems, human service agencies and systems, and social work practitioners	2.9	3.3	3.4
5.2 Can integrate knowledge of the current social welfare structures with the ability to analyze their impacts upon client systems, human service agencies and systems, and social work practitioners	2.9	3.3	3.4

Note. 4-point scale (1 = below expected, 2 = at expected, 3 = above expected, and 4 = exceptional); $^1N = 39$, $^2N = 20$, $^3N = 20$.

TABLE 4 Table Representing Field Supervisors Felt Students Demonstrated Competence on Policy Advocacy and Practice Behaviors (2012–2013), by Mean

EPAS Statement/Course Competency	2012–2013
2.1.1A Advocate for client access to services	3.1
2.1.5B Advocate for human rights & social/economic justice	3.1
2.1.8A Collaborate with colleagues & clients for policy action	3.1
2.1.9A Discover, appraise, and attend to changes to provide relevant services	3.0

Note. 4-point scale (1 = below expected, 2 = at expected, 3 = above expected, and 4 = exceptional), $N = 26$.

the profession. The increasing demonstration of competence also may have reflected that faculty were also improving their effectiveness at implementing the curriculum.

Evidence from student learning outcome surveys. The trend observed from the field supervisor evaluations was also recognized in feedback

TABLE 5 Table Representing Extent Students Felt They Mastered Policy Advocacy and Practice Objectives Fully and Mostly (2006–2011), by Range and 6-year Mean

Policy Advocacy and Practice Course Goal and Objective	6-Year Range	6-Year Mean
2.6 Define and discuss policy approaches/models	86–100%	92.4%
2.7 Examine and generate ideas about social welfare policy alternatives	90–100	95.2
2.8 Generate ideas for responses to policy-related injustices	86–96	91.7
2.9 Propose policy alternatives for selected agency level practice	87–100	95.3
2.10 Select professional ethical guidelines for policy formulation	91–100	97.0
3.11 Define and discuss policy advocacy strategies	87–100	93.7
3.12 Examine and propose advocacy strategies	87–100	95.7
3.13 Identify effective advocacy approaches	90–100	96.8
3.14 Design advocacy strategy for agency level practice	90–100	96.2
3.15 Select professional ethical guidelines to guide policy advocacy	87–100	95.8

Note. $N = 162$ out of 185 students.

TABLE 6 Table Representing Extent Students Felt They Mastered Policy Advocacy and Practice Objectives Fully or Mostly (2012–2013)

EPAS Statement/Course Competency	2-Year Range	2-Year Mean
2.1.1A Advocate for client access to services	91–100%	97%
2.1.5B Advocate for human rights & social/economic justice	100	100
2.1.8A Collaborate with colleagues & clients for policy action	95–100	96.7
2.1.9A Discover, appraise, and attend to changes to provide relevant services	95–100	98.3

Note. $N = 128$.

received from students. The data used to demonstrate the extent that students felt prepared to engage in policy advocacy and practice comes from the survey distributed to students at the end of their courses, *Measuring Achievement of Course Goals, Objectives and Outcomes*. Table 5 represents the data collected starting one year after the transition to the three-course policy sequence and was distributed at the conclusion of the Social Welfare Policy Practice course. The objectives and outcomes specific to advocacy and policy practice are reflected in these tables. One hundred eighty-five students completed the course between 2006 and 2011, with 162 (88%) responding to the course outcome survey. Table 6 reflects the course goals, objectives and outcomes after they were modified starting in fall 2012, similar to the field supervisor evaluations. During these two years, 128 students completed the course with 126 responding (98%) to the course outcome survey.

Under the previous policy-related course goals and after the students experienced the new sequence (Table 5), they rated their mastery over outcomes in a strongly positive manner. After the new EPAS was used to construct objectives (Table 6), their confidence in their skills appeared to be even stronger with higher levels of mastery noted by most students. Dramatic improvement occurred but the student outcome data also identified additional work needing to be done, such as generating ideas for responding to policy-related injustices (objective 2.8).

Evidence from recognition. Additional evidence of students' preparedness to participate in policy advocacy comes from recognition that they have received as a result of their work. For example, in 2012 a group of students completed a social welfare policy brief on the topic of expungement of felony records. They presented their brief and advocacy argument to the state assembly member of the district in which the University was located. The assembly member encouraged the students to continue their work and invited them to assist in eventually proposing legislative action on the topic. One of the students enrolled in a follow-up independent study course to continue their research; this research was selected to represent the University at the state capital for an event highlighting excellent undergraduate research projects. In the fall of 2013, one of the students continued to work with the state assembly member as part of an internship, assisting with the introduction of legislation on the topic of expungement of felony records. Other students were invited to provide testimony to the State Assembly.

Conclusion

After the shift to the three-course policy sequence and integration of experiential learning activities, the curriculum appears to have become more robust and effective in preparing undergraduate students to engage in policy practice and advocacy. Prior to the expanded curriculum, students and their field supervisors rated their policy advocacy and practice skills as barely adequate or an area of weakness. After the shift, both field supervisors and students have evaluated their competence typically above the level expected for BSW students; they are rated as having stronger mastery. The increased use of experiential learning activities along with the curriculum changes appears to be motivating students in successfully connecting their passions with policy advocacy. The program also continues to use the feedback to reflect on and enhance the policy curriculum.

Based on changes observed in student self-efficacy and supervisor perception, it seems appropriate to assume that these graduating social workers will be more likely than previous alumni to use their policy advocacy knowledge and skills to bring about social and economic justice for underserved and underrepresented groups. The significant social and economic issues facing the United States and other countries around the world demand this commitment from social workers.

Although this case study demonstrates favorable outcomes related to students preparedness to engage in policy advocacy and practice, further study is needed to determine the extent that this preparation is translating into practice once they are practicing social workers. As a program, we intend to facilitate a survey of alumni to determine the extent to which they are engaging in this critical aspect of social work practice. We would like to discern the extent to which their education and/or professional setting and norms are contributing to this engagement. As policy advocacy educators and practitioners, we look forward to furthering our investigation and analysis.

REFERENCES

Anderson, D. K., & Harris, B. M. (2005). Teaching social welfare policy: A comparison of two pedagogical approaches. *Journal of Social Work Education, 41*(3), 511–526. Retrieved from Expanded Academic ASAP.

Council on Social Work Education. (2008). *Educational policy and accreditation standards*. Alexandria, VA: CSWE.

de Chenu, L. (2012, July 8–12). Report on the "Joint World Conference on Social Work and Social Development: Action and Impact." Stockholm, Sweden: The Higher Education Academy.

Gal, J., & Weiss-Gal, I. (2013). *Social workers affecting social policy: An international perspective*. Chicago, IL: The University of Chicago Press.

Gibbons, J., & Gray, M. (2005). Teaching social work students about social policy. *Australian Social Work, 58*(1), 58–75. doi:10.1111/j.0312-407X.2005.00184.x

Heidemann, G., Fertig, R., Jansson, B., & Kim, H. (2011). Practicing policy, pursuing change, and promoting social justice: A policy instructional approach. *Journal of Social Work Education, 47*(1), 37–52. doi:10.5175/JSWE.2010.2010.200800118

Henman, P. (2012). Making social policy "sexy": Evaluating a teaching innovation. *Australian Social Work, 65*(3), 341–354. Retrieved from Yeshiva University Libraries.

Hoefer, R. (2013). Policy practice in social work: The United States. In Gal, J. & Weiss-Gal, I. (Eds.), *Social workers affecting social policy: An international perspective* (pp. 161–182). Bristol, UK: Policy Press.

Holmberg-Herrstrom, E. (2012, July 8) Joint World Conference on Social Work and Social Development. Stockholm, Sweden Opening remarks.

National Association of Social Workers. (2008). NASW Code of Ethics (Guide to the Everyday Professional Conduct of Social Workers). Washington, DC: NASW.

Rocha, C. J. (2000). Evaluating experiential teaching methods in a policy practice course: The case for service learning to increase political participation. *Journal of Social Work Education, 36*(1), 53–63.

Weiss, I., Gal, J., & Katan, J. (2006). Social policy for social work: A teaching agenda. *British Journal of Social Work, 36*(5), 789–806.

Index

Abell, N. 146
Abramovitz, M. 8, 145
active learning 147, 148
Almog-Bar, M. 29
Amnesty International 119
Anderson, D.K. 11, 22, 92, 94, 95, 149, 170, 172
Andrews, A.B. 105
anti-personnel mines 122–3
Argentina 114
Association for Public Policy Analysis and Management (APPAM) 147
Australia 148

Banning, S.A. 51
Bar-Zuri, R. 21
Barusch, A.S. 113
Bass, G.D. 49, 50, 58
Bayefsky, A.F. 118
Beimers, D. 105
Bernal, Jorge 118–19
Bernklau Halvor, C.D. 92
Berry, J.M. 29, 30, 49–50
Bessell, S. 119
Blackwood, A. 29
Bogo, M. 146
Boris, E.T. 49, 50
Borrie, J. 122
Bortree, D.S. 51
Brabant, S. 122
Bromfield, N.F. 113
Bruning, S.D. 51, 62
Bryant, A. 31
Buechler, S. 71
Butler, A.C. 146
Butler, S.S. 95, 105
Byers, K. 105

Cameron, K.S. 31, 32
Cameron, M.A. 122
Canary, D.J. 51, 52

Caputo, R.K. 115, 131, 132
case advocacy 117, 118
case study 169–82; influence of accrediting body and professional organizations 171–2; responses to increased need for teaching social welfare policy advocacy 172–3; social policy advocacy instruction in US and abroad 170–1; US baccalaureate 173–82
Center for Justice and International Law 118
Chandler, M.A. 149
Chapin, R.K. 119
children 131, 147, 152; Child Rights International Network 119; views of 120
Christie, L. 149
civic engagement and civic literacy 128–42; discussion 139–41; literature review 129–33; methods 133–5; results 135–8
Civic Voluntarism Theory 10
Clark, E.J. 145
Clark, M. 74
class 146
clinical practice 131, 132, 145, 147
Clinton, Bill 114–15
cluster munitions 122–3
Cobb, D. 2
Cochran, G. 7
codes of ethics 170; NASW 141, 145, 171–2
Colby, I.C. 8, 97
Comartin, E. 70
Comerford, S.A. 105
Competing Values Framework (CVF) *see* electronic advocacy, Open Systems model and internal structures
Convention on the Elimination of All Forms of Discrimination Against Women 118
Convention on the Elimination of All Forms of Racial Discrimination 118
cost-benefit analysis 115
Council on Social Work Education (CSWE) 93, 94, 131, 145, 147, 153, 171, 172, 174, 176; human rights 112, 115, 117, 119, 123

INDEX

Creswell, J. 74
Cummins, L.K. 7, 113, 117, 145

Davidson, J.S. 118
Davis, G. 71
de Chenu, L. 170
De Vita, C. 30
Defeis, E.F. 114
deKieffer, D.E. 50, 60, 61
democratic participation 142; civic literacy 132–4, 137–8, 140, 142; voting in elections 8, 130, 131, 132, 135–7, 140
DeRigne, L. 92, 95, 106, 141
Dewey, J. 147
diabetes 152
Dillman, D.A. 33
DiNitto, D.M. 113
disabilities: Disability Rights International (formerly Mental Disability Rights International) 118–19; participation 120
discrimination 118, 145
Docherty, B. 122
Dochy, F. 148
Donaldson, L.P. 30, 51, 52–3
Dozier, D.M. 51

e-mail: NASW chapters and communication with members 97, 98, 103
Edelenbos, J. 61
education see students and policy practice
Educational Policy and Accreditation Standards (EPAS) 112, 123, 171, 176, 181
Edwards, B. 71
Edwards, H.R. 96
electronic advocacy, Open systems model and internal structures 27–44; discussion 43; future directions, future study 44; limitations 43–4; literature review 29–33; method 33–6; results 36–42; study purpose 28–9
electronic advocacy and social work member groups and coalitions 96
electronic outreach 81
Ellis, R.A. 8
environmental issues 139
ethics, codes of 141, 145, 170, 171–2
ethnicity 133
European Commission of Human Rights 118
evidence-based policy practice 152
experiential learning 144–62; case study 169–82; discussion and implications 160–2; diving below the headlines 149–53; from social policy to policy practice 147–9; meaning of policy practice 145; methods 153–5; results 155–60; study limitations 160; teaching policy practice in social work 146–7
Ezell, M. 8, 10, 22, 92, 94

Figueira-McDonough, J. 145
Finn, P. 70
fire deaths among children, house 152
Fisher, R. 129, 146
Fitzgerald, E. 30–1, 92
Freeman, E.M. 147
Frumkin, P. 49, 50
Furrow, B.R. 117

Gable, L. 116–17
Gal, J. 8, 9, 12, 21, 170, 171
Gallagher, A. 114
Gammonley, D. 118
Gamson, J. 86
Garrahan, P. 32
Geiger, B. 69
Gen, S. 49, 64
Generation X 130
Germany, J.B. 31
Gibbons, J. 148, 170, 171, 172
Gibelman, M. 30
Gifford, B.D. 32
Glaser, B. 74
Glater, J.D. 149
Global Agenda for Social Action 170
Global Standards for Social Work Education and Training 145–6
grassroots advocacy 52
Greene, R. 7
Greenhalgh, R.G. 31
growth rate of nonprofit sector 28
Grubesic, T. 69
Grunig, J.E. 51
Guo, C. 29

Hager, M.A. 33, 44
Hamilton, D. 8, 92, 94, 107
Handicap International 123
Hartnell, C.A. 31
Hartnett, H. 8, 93, 97
Hauser, S.M. 131, 132, 133
Haynes, K.S. 113, 117
health care 115–17; diabetes 152; public health and education 147
Healy, L.M. 111, 117
Heidemann, G. 170
Henman, P. 172
Hessenius, B. 50
Hillman, A.A. 118
Hmelo-Silver, C.E. 148
Hoefer, R. 8, 61, 70, 96, 104, 106, 117, 128, 145, 170, 171, 172
Hokenstad, M.C.T. 115
Holmberg-Herrstrom, E. 170
home foreclosures 152
Hon, L.C. 51, 52, 53, 54, 55, 56, 63

INDEX

house fire deaths among children 152
human rights and social work curriculum 111–23, 145, 171; collaboration 119–23; policy advocacy 117–19, 123; policy analysis 115–17, 123; policy formulation 113–15, 123
Human Rights Watch 119, 122
human trafficking 113–15, 175
Hundley, W. 1, 2
Hymans, D. 146, 147, 150

Iatridis, D.S. 145
immigration 152
impact analysis 115
indigenous peoples 119, 121, 133, 175
Inter-American Commission on Human Rights 118–19
International Association of Schools of Social Work 112, 145–6
International Committee of the Red Cross 119
International Covenant on Civil and Political Rights 118
International Covenant on Economic, Social and Cultural Rights: right to health 115–16
International Federation of Social Workers 111, 145–6; Statement of Ethical Principles 141
international and national human rights policy 113–15, 123
Israel, legislative advocacy in 7–24; conceptual basis 9–11; discussion 20–4; findings 16–20; method 12–16
Israeli schools of social work 148–9

Jackson-Elmoore, C. 96
Jacobson, W.B. 8
Jansson, B.S. 7, 113, 115, 117, 145, 149
Jenkins, P. 71
Johnson, A.K. 145
joint advocacy 53
Joint World Conference on Social Work and Social Development 170

Kahne, J. 133
Kalliath, T.J. 32
Kanter, B. 31
Karger, H.J. 113
Keeter, S. 129, 130, 131, 134, 140
Khazanchi, S. 31
Ki, E.J. 51, 52, 54
Kiesler, S. 32
Kilbane, T. 93, 97, 106
Kimberlin, S.E. 29
King, N. 32
Kingdon, J. 71, 73, 85
Kleinfield, N.R. 149
Kline, R.B. 57
Klinenberg, E. 150

Koestler, A. 132
Kolb, A. 148
Kovacs, R. 49, 50, 53, 60, 61
Kriesi, H. 81, 84

Lane, S.R. 97
Lawrence, K.A. 32
leadership 30
Ledingham, J.A. 50, 62
legislative advocacy 117; Israel 7–24; lobbying *see separate entry*; NASW involvement in 92–108
legislative advocacy in Israel 7–24; conceptual basis 9–11; discussion 20–4; facilitation 10, 22, 23, 24; findings 16–20; method 12–16; motivation 10–11, 22–3, 24; opportunity 9, 21–2, 23, 24; policy practice training 11, 14, 17, 22–4
legislative advocacy, NASW involvement in 92–108; barriers to advocacy 105–6; discussion 103–7; implications for social work education 106–7; legislative advocacy days 97, 99, 100, 101–3, 104, 105–6, 107; literature review 93–7; method 98; NASW chapters 96–7; professional members 94, 98–9, 103, 104, 105, 107; purpose of study 93; results 98–103; social work students 94–5, 97, 99–101, 102, 104–8
Lens, V. 117
Leon, C. 70, 71, 86
Levenson, J. 68, 69, 70
Lewin, K. 3
Lewis, C. 70
Linhorst, D.M. 147
lobbying 8, 49, 53, 158; Lobby/Legislative Advocacy Days 97, 99, 100, 101–3, 104, 105–6, 107, 117, 141, 175; sex offender rights organizations 73, 80–1; Undergraduate Day at the State Capitol (URDC) 152–3
Logan, W. 69, 70
Lombe, M. 63
Lyons, J. 132, 133

McAdam, D. 71, 72
McCarthy, J. 71
Macindoe, H. 29
McNutt, J. 30, 34, 35, 36
McPhail, C. 72
Manalo, V. 92, 95, 105, 106, 117
Mancini, C. 70
Mary, N.L. 131, 132
Medicaid 117
Medina, C. 118
Mellinger, M.S. 50, 63
Mendes, P. 7
'middle classization' 146
migrant workers 120–1

INDEX

minimum wage 153
Mosley, J. 7, 9, 29, 49, 53
Muthén, L.K. 60

Nadkarni, V.V. 117
Nah, S. 29
Nash, T. 123
NASW involvement in legislative advocacy 92–108; barriers to advocacy 105–6; chapters of NASW 96–7; discussion 103–7; implications for social work education 106–7; literature review 93–7; method 98; purpose of study 93; results 98–103
National Association of Social Workers (NASW) 147, 172; civic engagement of members 131; Code of Ethics 141, 145, 171–2; involvement in legislative advocacy 92–108; meaning of policy practice 145
networking 51, 52, 53, 56, 57, 58–9, 60, 61; sex offender rights organizations 71, 81, 86
neuroscience 147
Newman, M. 73
Nicholson-Crotty, 57
non-governmental organizations (NGOs) 119, 122, 123
Nuckles, C.R. 148

Obama, Barack 130
O'Connor, M.K. 115
older persons 150; participation in decision-making 120
Open Systems model, internal structures and electronic advocacy 27–44; discussion 43; future directions, future study 44; limitations 43–4; literature review 29–33; method 33–6; results 36–42; study purpose 28–9
opportunity theory, political *see* sex offender rights organizations
O'Reilly, T. 31
organizational culture 21; definition 31; engagement with advocacy activities: effect of 27–44
organizational emergence *see* sex offender rights organizations
organizational-public relationships (OPRs) *see* relationship management
Ostroff, C. 32

Padgett, D. 76
Paraguay 118–19
Park, H. 51, 53, 61
participation in decision-making 119–23; *see also* civic engagement and civic literacy
Patient Protection and Affordable Care Act 116–17
Patterson, M.G. 33, 34, 35, 36, 39

Peters, A. 122
Pierce, D. 7, 8
Policy Practice Engagement (PPE) framework 7–24; discussion 20–4; facilitation 10, 22, 23, 24; findings 16–20; method 12–16; motivation 10–11, 22–3, 24; opportunity 9, 21–2, 23, 24; policy practice training 11, 14, 17, 22–4
political engagement *see* civic engagement and civic literacy
political opportunity theory *see* sex offender rights organizations
Pollack, D. 117
Portney, K.E. 131
Powell, J.Y. 92, 95, 117
public health and education 147
Putnam, R.D. 130

Quinn, R.E. 32, 33

Reich, R. 129
Reichert, E. 111, 115
Reisman, J. 72
relationship building: characteristic of effective advocacy 268; relationship management 48–64; and sex offender rights organizations 80, 85
relationship management 48–64; access 51, 53, 55, 57, 58, 59–60, 61; aims of study 53; assurances 51, 52, 53, 56, 57, 58, 59, 60–1; discussion 60–4; implications for practitioners 61–2; implications for research 62–3; methods 54–8; networking 51, 52, 53, 56, 57, 58–9, 60, 61; openness 51–2, 53, 55, 57, 58, 59–60, 61; organizational-public relationships (OPRs) 50–1; policy advocacy as human service administrative activity 49–50; positivity 51, 53, 56, 57, 58–9; results 58–60; sharing of tasks 51, 52–3, 55–6, 57, 58, 59, 60, 61, 62
Richan, W.C. 53, 60
Ritter, J.A. 7, 8, 23, 92, 94, 105, 107, 129, 131, 133, 142
Roark, C. 1, 2
Rocha, C. 8, 22, 92, 95, 145, 147, 148, 172
Roeger, K. 28
Rome, S.H. 49, 92, 94, 131, 132, 141–2
Rotela, Julio César 118–19
Rothenberg, L. 72
Rothman, J. 145, 146
Rubin, A. 73, 146
Rubinstein, A. 9
Ruggiano, N. 49, 50, 54, 57, 61

Saidel, J.R. 30
Salamon, L.M. 50
Salcido, R.M. 93, 96, 97
Sargeant, A. 51, 61

INDEX

Saulnier, C.F. 95
Saunders, E. 68
Scanlon, E. 93, 97
Schachter, H.L. 29
Schein, E.H. 31
Schneider, R.L. 9, 117
Schorr, L.B. 152
Secker, E. 119
Segal, E.A. 113
Semple, K. 149
Sewpaul, V. 146
sex offender rights organizations 67–87; anti-SORN movement and social movement organizations (SMOs) 70–3; coalition building 73, 81, 86; constitutional challenges to SORN policies 70, 72, 83; discussion 84–7; electronic outreach 81; future studies 87; media 68, 73, 75, 80, 81, 82, 83, 84, 85–6; methods 73–6; networking 71, 81, 86; organizational emergence 71–2, 76–80; political opportunities 72–3, 81–4, 85, 86; proactive 76, 78–86, 87; professional membership 79, 84–5, 86; reactive 76, 78–86, 87; research and policy analysis 81, 86; results 76–84; (organizational emergence) 76–80; (tactics) 80–4; sex offender registration and notification (SORN) policies 69–70; testimony 73, 81, 86
Sherraden, M.S. 53, 148
Shrout, P.E. 60
Skinner, R.M. 49, 50, 53, 60, 61
Skocpol, T. 130, 131
Smith, S.R. 29
social media 29, 30–1, 36, 37, 43, 73, 98
social movement organizations (SMOs) *see* sex offender rights organizations
Social Work Day at United Nations 117–18
Sommers, B.D. 117
Specht, H. 129, 131, 145
Steen, J.A. 111
Sternberg, S. 149
Stolz, B.A. 114, 115
Strauss, A. 75
student debt 152
student-focused learning 147, 148
students and policy practice 94–5; case study 169–82; civic engagement and civic literacy 128–42; experiential learning 144–62, 169–82; Global Standards for Social Work Education and Training 145–6; human rights and social work curriculum 111–23; state chapters of NASW 94–5, 97, 99–101, 102, 104–8

Suárez, D.F. 30, 49
Sumariwalla, R.D. 33

Tabachnick, B.G. 56, 57
Tarrow, S. 71, 72, 86
teaching *see* students and policy practice
Teater, B. 50, 52, 61, 85, 87, 96
Teitelbaum, J. 117
Terry, K. 69
Teush, O. 14
Tewksbury, R. 68, 69, 70
theory in advocacy research, role of 3–4
Tilly, C. 72
Torture Convention 118
Tower, L.E. 11, 22, 94, 95, 105
trafficking, human 113–15, 175
Tredinnick, L. 31

Undergraduate Day at the State Capitol (URDC) 152–3
United Nations: Economic and Social Council 116; General Assembly 115; human rights 113–16, 117–18; Social Work Day 117–18

van Dijk, P. 118
Van Horn, C. 70
van Wormer, K. 115
Verba, S. 10, 14
volunteerism 8, 130, 131, 134, 135, 137, 139, 140, 141
voting in elections 8, 130, 131, 132, 135–7, 140

Walz, T. 146
Weaver, R.D. 94
Weiss, I. 94, 146, 148, 170
Weiss-Gal, I. 9, 10, 22, 148
welfare state and social workers 129, 142
West, M.A. 32
Whitaker, T. 147
Whittier, N. 71
Witkin, S.L. 111
Wolk, J.L. 94, 150
Wronka, J. 111
Wyers, N.L. 145

Zafft, C. 32
Zald, M. 71, 72
Zammuto, R.F. 32
Zubrzycki, J. 11
Zull, J.E. 147